PARENTISH

—·—

THE ULTIMATE PARENTS' HANDBOOK ON PUBERTY FOR GIRLS AND BOYS

LONDON FORD

Contents

CONTENTS

INTRODUCTION

Parents can only give good advice or put them on the right paths, but the final forming of a person's character lies in their own hands. –Anne Frank

Kids will always complain that you just don't get them and that you don't know what it's like for them. To them, you are an adult, a parent who has no idea about their struggles or about what it's like to be in their shoes. They quite easily can't comprehend or forget that you, too, were once a kid or that you had the same troubles as them. But remember when you were a kid and thought the same. This is the eternal loop of the generation gap. Why the problems seem relatable to you and so foreign to them is that while you have survived your teenage years, they are living theirs. So they are entitled to their share of moodiness and sleepiness...and all those troubles that this weird time brings for us humans.

Parents Do Not Understand Their Children

Most teens complain about their parents not understanding them because of the "generation gap." It was rare in the past because women used to marry at a young age. As a result, the generation gap was as wide as it is today. Today, the majority of parents (both) work. As a result, they can only sometimes meet the child's emotional needs. Parents must recognize that times have changed. Today's children are very open about everything. Children are more advanced as a result of the internet. Parents must understand that for their children to compete, they must be aware of all advancements.

It Is Also Not Always Appropriate to Blame the Parents

Children today have high expectations, thanks to technological advancements and liberal ideas. When a child is young, he expects to have the most recent games. He expects to have the latest bikes and so on as he grows. It is only sometimes possible for parents to understand their child's needs. Children today are more liberal as a result of media and television. Almost all social issues are widely known. Children should understand that it is unfair to expect parents to always understand them, knowing they are from a different generation. It all comes down to how the child is raised in the end. Children cannot be blamed if they are exposed to violence, divorce, and financial difficulties from a young age. A child needs to be properly nurtured.

Maybe you feel some of the following things:

- You're scared of slowly losing your child as they step into the secrecy-led years of adolescence.

- You're scared that you're not doing a good job of raising your teens.

- You feel guilty for working and not being there for your teen more often.

- You don't know how to talk to your kids about all of this and are worried that whatever you say to them will not mean as much to them.

- You feel like you don't know the right words for topics such as sex and pregnancy.

By the time you finish reading this book, you'll understand

- how to help your teen learn about their body and the changes they are experiencing.

- connecting and effectively communicating with your teen

- how to make your teen feel confident.

- how to make your teen be accepted.

- answering questions from your kids.

- how to be relevant in your kids' growth journey

- how to help your teenager grow through puberty and its changes.

This book is a single one-point source to help you teach your kids what puberty is and the changes associated with it.

Chapter 1: P: Pushing Past the Enigma

Does your teenager always ask for privacy? Do they have a sign outside their room saying, "Please knock" or "No trespassing" or "Do not enter without permission?" What do these signs mean? Why does your teenager want this wall between you and them?

The most significant trouble as a parent of growing teenagers is to see them pull away from you instead of coming straight to you like they did when they were younger. They don't precisely make talking to them so easy, do they? But the question is, why do they do this? Why do they behave so distant? Is it normal? Should you do anything about it? Should you not?

It is reasonable for you to worry about any abrupt changes a 13-year-old may experience, especially regarding teens and privacy. Your adolescent daughter is probably in her room at this specific time to feel more independent and in charge of her life. As she begins to experience physical changes, privacy may become increasingly crucial. However, we could think endlessly about why your adolescent daughter requests more seclusion. Asking the question directly is the greatest method to get the answer.

What Causes Teenagers to Be So Distant From Their Parents?

Teenagers' relationships with their family and friends undergo significant changes as they experience physical and mental development. Family relationships frequently change as a child reaches puberty. Teenagers desire greater independence and emotional separation from their parents. Teens frequently switch focus to friendships and social interactions. This applies to friends of the same gender, friends in the same gender groups, and friends in cross-gender groups. Interest in dating and intimate relationships is sparked by sexual maturity.

Relationships With Oneself Change

The teenage years are when one comes to a new sense of who they are. This might entail changes to these self-perceptions:

Independence

This entails taking charge of one's affairs and acting according to one's reasoning and judgment. Teenagers begin to learn how to solve issues on their own. Teenagers begin to assume additional responsibilities as their capacity for reasoning and intuition grows. They begin to take pleasure in their ideas and deeds. Teenagers also begin to think about and fantasize about adulthood (for instance, college or job training, work, and marriage).

Identity

This is referred to as one's personality or sense of self. The development of a strong sense of personal identity is among the main goals of adolescence. A teen becomes accustomed to and accepts a physically more mature physique. Additionally, they develop their capacity for independent judgment and decision-making. The teen begins to build a sense of who they are when these things happen, and they confront their issues. When a teen cannot resolve conflicts over their identification as a physically, sexually, and independently capable person, problems with forming a distinct sense of self or identity arise.

Self-Esteem

This is the way you feel about yourself. The response to the question "How much do I like myself?" will reveal your level of self-esteem. A decline in self-esteem at the outset of adolescence is rather typical. This results from different physical changes, new ideas, and novel thoughts. Teenagers are now self-aware and deliberate about their goals. They observe discrepancies between their behavior and their beliefs. Teenagers must decide how they view themselves once they consider their behaviors and traits. Teenagers frequently value physical appearance. Teens frequently suffer from low self-esteem when they don't feel attractive in their own eyes. Self-esteem typically rises when teenagers get a greater understanding of who they are.

Change in Peer Relationships

Teenagers socialize more with their peers. They claim that their friends have made them feel more accepted and understood. Spending time with parents and other family members is decreasing.

Teens with similar interests, social classes, and cultural backgrounds tend to form close connections. Teen friendships broaden to encompass similarities in attitudes, values, and shared activities, whereas childhood friendships typically focus on shared activities. Teen friendships can frequently stem from shared academic interests. The exploration of identities and the definition of one's sense of self are aided, especially for girls, by deep, personal, and self-disclosing talks with friends. Teenagers can explore their sexuality and feelings through conversations with their close friends. Teenage boy friendships are frequently less close than those of girls.

Male-Female Relationships Change

Sexual attraction, societal and cultural expectations, and influences impact the change in male-female and sexual relationships. In male-female or sexual relationships, social and cultural norms and behaviors are learned via experience and observation. Developmental challenges during adolescence include attempting to restrain aggressive and sexual drives. Finding potential or genuine romantic partnerships also happens. Impulsive conduct, various experimental encounters of mutual exploring, and eventually sexual contact are all possible sexual activities during adolescence. Males and females have different expectations of romantic and sexual relationships due to biological differences and disparities in how they interact in society. These could affect sexual encounters and possibly impact future sexual behavior and relationships. It may be possible to find a sexual partnership that is mutually pleasant over time.

Changes in Family Connections

Separating from one's family as a young adult and being independent is one of the developmental objectives of adolescence. Coming to grips with one's sentiments regarding one's family is a step in this process. Teenagers begin to understand during adolescence that their parents and other significant adults don't always know everything or have the answers to all their problems. It's typical and acceptable for some teenagers to rebel against their parents. Disagreements frequently get smaller with time. However, compared to fathers, relationships with moms may undergo more change. Teenagers are more inclined to ask their peers for assistance as they become more self-reliant concerning their parents.

Does Your Boy Not Talk?

My son was hilarious and loving when he was younger. He loved to ask questions and had a ton of them. He was reserved with individuals he didn't know well, but he was animated and entertaining around his relatives and friends. Very little about his day, dreams, friends, and aspirations were unknown to me.

Then middle school started. He first grew large and ungainly and began to smell like a teenager. I anticipated those modifications. But I expected his personality to remain the same. My once-sweet and talkative son was giving me the silent treatment at the age of 14. He answered questions in the barest of terms and never posed any of his own. He seldom left his room. If he spoke at all, it was with a sulky and nasty attitude. In other words, he was making a fantastic impression of every representation of teenage guys I'd ever seen who gathered weapons and then went on murderous rampages. He frightened me. Why do teen boys cut off the conversation? Was his lack of speech signaling that he was about to lose it?

Tongue-Tied by Hormones

Miles Groth, a psychology professor at Wagner College and the creator of the Boys to Men blog on Psychology Today, says, "Becoming silent has been the response of freshly pubescent boys since the species began." It's nothing new, he continued. "[It's] not relevant to the present or to happenings right now."

He noted that boys go through many bodily changes at this age. According to Groth, "They are very self-conscious, evaluating the way that adults, peers, and members of the opposing sex, or in some cases the same sex, are perceived of them." They are less inclined to commit themselves verbally because of their self-consciousness.

According to Dr. John Duffy, author of *The Available Parent: Expert Advice for Raising Successful, Resilient, and Connected Teens and Tweens,* middle school marks the beginning of adolescence for most boys and the ensuing social uneasiness. "The less stated, the less one is subject to mockery. The quiet serves as a form of self-defense in this way.

It's natural for worried parents to imagine the worst, as I did automatically, but the odds are strong that a kid in his adolescence is silent. It signifies the profound physical and psychological changes brought on by puberty. According to Duffy, "Most males grow out of this phase with little harm done." From a parent's perspective, it might be intimidating and frightening because silence can be interpreted as insulating or even depressive. Make sure your middle school son is doing okay by periodically checking in with him. But remember that his quiet is probably within the range of normal development.

According to Katey McPherson, executive director of The Gurian Institute and co-author of the book *Why Teens Fail: What To Fix,* even my son's reserved responses to my questions are typical of many boys as they mature into men. She notes that women have more significant connective tissue between the right and left brains. "Compared to men, we process language far more quickly. I believe that women verbally abuse their male partners."

Groth suggests that rather than reacting to this specific change in many boys' temperaments out of fear, we can start by focusing on what is going right. Has your son got any interests? Does he enjoy hanging out with friends? Does he appear to be interested in interacting with others? If the answer is affirmative, it indicates that his new monosyllabic speech pattern is typical.

Of course, if he won't talk, it could be challenging to find out this information. However, it may not be that he won't speak as much as he is having a verbal block due to his present hormone crisis, particularly when Mom keeps peppering him with questions in response to the few words he gets to squeak out. Take him for a stroll, advises McPherson. Make him move. And ask him a question or two at a time.

Long, honest chats may need to wait for a time, but keeping up with his life online is another method to be informed. Because teens' lives take place on social media, parents should always watch how their children use Twitter, Facebook, Instagram, and other sites. Ask him about today's events on Twitter, what social media platform his buddies are using, or for a hilarious Vine video. While figuring out his social media habits, you will discover more about him.

Negative Aspects of Being Quiet

It's time to pay notice—and get treatment—if your son withdraws from his classmates, displays despondency, or uses or abuses drugs or alcohol. Someone who is depressed believes there is no escape. They believe they are in a hopeless situation and that there is no way out.

In general, girls are more likely to be forthright about sharing their feelings when they are hurt. However, because they are more likely to clam up, guys who are depressed may go unnoticed entirely. According to Groth, four times as many teenage boys commit suicide as teenage girls. "Not speaking with you is pretty common. I would be more concerned if he also refused to communicate with his peers, people outside the home, or anyone else."

Eventually, my son broke his silence. The trip was long and unsettling, littered with indicators that he was having depressing thoughts. He made suicidal threats, withdrew from social interactions, and hid in his room. I sought treatment for him after taking his threats seriously. Together, we went through it. We both made mistakes. I was pretty explicit about the fact that he was loved and that he wasn't the first adolescent to experience this. He eventually recovered, much like someone with a protracted, debilitating flu. My son is once again talkative, verbose, humorous, and willing to share his dreams and observations at age 20. Again, we are friends.

How Can You Help?

Emotional distance is regarded as typical behavior as a teenager matures through adolescence. This is the evolution of adolescents discovering their independence and figuring out how to handle their problems. Parents should consider teens acting distantly as a chronic problem that can be resolved. Realistic expectations, scenario analysis, and solution-finding are crucial for boosting parent and teen involvement.

Many parents lament that their adolescent is skipping out on family events, staying in their rooms, or using their telephones excessively, among other things. These may be the initial indications that they are bothered by a deeper problem. The ability of the parent and teen to communicate can be hampered if this distant conduct is not adequately addressed. Both modest and significant internal problems in the teen can serve as causes for distant behavior. Teenagers frequently face challenges, including peer conflicts, bullying, and academic difficulties. Depression, drug use, alcohol abuse, and severe bullying are more serious problems that can lead to a kid becoming emotionally distant. Teenagers occasionally worry that their parents won't comprehend what they are going through or that they will let them down.

Don'ts when dealing with a reclusive teen:

- Don't begin to nag your teen about contributing more to the household dynamic.

- Don't put penalties on them as a threat.

- Don't ask repeated questions.

- Don't show your rage or hatred at them.

Here are some pointers to help you connect with your teenager who is emotionally distant:

Speak Their Language

Speak to your teen in their preferred manner (e.g., email, text message, instant message, or a non-embarrassing post on their favorite social media website). Even though it seems impersonal to you, it can be simpler for him to discuss delicate topics with you on the internet without physically seeing you.

Be in the Same Spot at the Same Time

You and your teen will have something to do together that isn't too stressful if you make supper together every night or at least once a week. Any household work or routine activity that allows you to spend time together but doesn't need much thought or conversation can foster a relaxed environment where your adolescent can open up to you, even if the chat is about unrelated topics. Teenagers are more likely to feel at ease speaking with you when they don't have to look at you, like while driving.

Talk About Movies

Sharing your taste in movies with your adolescent is another way to strengthen your relationship, whether you're talking about an old favorite or one of today's trendiest flicks.

Don't Lead Your Teen Astray

Your teen is sometimes in the wrong because she prefers to approach things differently. For instance, even though most parents want their teenagers to attend college, they might not be interested. Instead of being shocked if your kid decides against attending college, try to reach a compromise. She might be able to balance working and studying part-time. She could go to a technical school rather than pursue a general degree. Teenagers can sometimes grow significantly by letting go a little.

Say Something Good About Them

Tell your adolescent at least one good thing about him daily to help him develop positive self-esteem. To foster a positive self-image, ask him to add something more to your list that he likes or feels confident about.

Spend Time With Your Teen and Her Closest Pals

Take her and one or two of her closest pals shopping, to a fun class (e.g., pottery, jewelry making, cooking), or for pedicures. As long as you don't interfere, finding a shared pastime with your adolescent's buddies will probably win you some points with everyone.

Delegate Some Authority to Your Adolescent

As a parent, you might wonder how reconnecting with your adolescent by giving her some responsibilities can help. Giving your teen responsibility around the house demonstrates your faith in her if appropriately done and without coming off as a directive or an order. If she has just received her license, it can be as straightforward as going to the post office or picking up her younger sister after school. She thinks you consider her a young woman today when you make small, responsible gestures. This will make you feel proud of yourself and grateful for continuing to put more and more trust in her.

Leave Your Teen Alone

Any relationship will occasionally benefit from some distance. Being in charge of someone else or trying to force them to see things your way won't help. Your teen will likely seek you out if you offer her the chance to do so if you take some time to yourself, step away, and keep things informal.

Offer Support

Support her by attending her sessions, performances, or sporting events. She might not recognize your presence, but she probably wants you there to offer support—as long as you don't make her uncomfortable.

Be Available

So that your teen knows where to find you if and when she needs to talk, hang out in a common area of your home, or develop a schedule where you are available at the same time each day or on the same night each week.

Arrange an Activity Together

Each month, arrange at least one outing or activity for you and your adolescent. Plan the activity in pairs so that he has some say in what you do. Give him a spending and time limit, and let him decide where you go and what you do. You can get to know each other's interests better this way, which may surprise you both.

Allow Your Teen to Drive on a Little Road Trip

This is ideal for teenagers who have just received their driver's licenses. Any exciting location of your adolescent's choice works for an afternoon of bonding, regardless of the destination. It might be as simple as scheduling regular driving practice sessions in the countryside or on city streets to help your kid improve her driving abilities.

Request Hugs Occasionally

Although he might sigh and roll his eyes, your child is likely secretly happy. Let it go if he doesn't seem interested. He will be aware that the offer is still available. Family members used to question why I allowed this big child to cling to me in such a way, but I understood that it was his method of intimacy.

Your Child Can Benefit From Emotional Distance

The teen years are characterized by investigations into identity, autonomy, and independence outside the family system. Perhaps children would prefer to spend more time in their rooms. They will believe their buddies comprehend them much better than their parents. They will distance themselves from their parents. It cannot be very pleasant for parents.

Your youngster is not the only one affected by this shift. Yes, this is how your adolescent is acquiring adult skills. Psychologists refer to this process as individuation, which, despite being upsetting for parents, is natural and beneficial for your child. While it may make you uncomfortable as a parent, your child's growing independence from you marks their entry into the adult world. It is hoped that they will use the talents you have taught them in their lives as young people.

If you think your child's behavior changes are abnormal, consult your pediatrician. Sudden behavioral changes can also be caused by depression, bullying, substance misuse, and other circumstances.

Emotional Distance Is Not an Excuse for Abuse

Remember that just because your child is letting go of the closeness he formerly shared with you doesn't mean he has the right to treat you disrespectfully. Additionally, he is not permitted to disregard the regulations of the home. Healthy emotional distance is letting your child be independent and even encouraging it but still holding them responsible for following your household's norms and expectations.

Remind yourself that your child's requirements for alone time and time with friends are developmental while dealing with the developmental needs of a teenager. Maintain a definite and precise set of expectations. And try your best to encourage her growth.

Self-Care Is Important

Take good care of yourself. Losing a younger kid to adulthood causes significant anguish for parents. Permit yourself to be depressed and unhappy. And if you are having problems letting go, try not to be too hard on yourself. Both children and parents are learning as they make the transition to maturity.

Check out James Lehman's essay on *Sudden Changes In Children* for more information on this topic. He discusses rapid behavioral changes that might be an indication of a more severe problem while doing an excellent job of explaining individuation and providing some valuable tools.

Undoubtedly, this is a challenging aspect of parenting. But we should allow our children the freedom to discover who they are in a respectful and safe environment.

Segue: The next chapter will talk about responsibility, giving it, and taking it.

CHAPTER 2: A: ACTING RESPONSIBLY

Teenagers are always asking to be treated like an adult. They keep complaining that they are not a child anymore, right? Well, they are. Not completely, but to an extent. They need to feel like they are contributing too; they need to feel important. If they don't get that sense of importance and fulfillment at home, they will seek it outside. It's better that, as a parent, you start recognizing their potential and teach them a few lessons in responsibility, contributions, and accountability. Lessons learned now stay with them forever, modeling their behavior as an adult. But be cautious. Children learn from what we do, not from what we say should be done.

Why Is Giving Responsibilities to Your Teenager a Good Idea?

Being "accountable" means accepting responsibility for one's actions; every parent wants their teen to exhibit this quality. Children develop as considerate people and responsible citizens when parents inculcate a sense of personal responsibility for their decisions and actions. Teenagers who don't take responsibility point the finger at others, break the law because they think it's unfair, and make excuses for their behavior no matter how it affects others.

Why do so many teenagers and young people lack this vital quality if we all want to produce responsible teenagers? Establishing accountability is a difficult task. It's a drawn-out procedure that calls for tact and patience. It will often seem our efforts are in vain, which might lead some parents to give up. But have courage! It is possible to raise responsible kids in today's world, and if you persevere, you will eventually watch your teen grow into a responsible adult.

Techniques to Teach Your Teenagers Responsibility

Here are some techniques you can apply to teach your teen to be responsible.

Display Personal Accountability

The best method for parents to teach their teens anything is through role modeling. Embody whatever value you wish your teen to possess by doing it yourself. Therefore, you should act responsibly if you want your adolescent to do so. Do not assign blame. Follow the rules, and don't try to escape the penalties for breaking them. If you make a mistake, own up to it, and say you're sorry. Leave a note, for instance, if you accidentally hit the door of the car next to you in the parking lot.

Make Responsibility a Priority in Your Household

Your family's culture represents your values, norms, expectations, and aspirations. Each family member must take responsibility for their actions and behaviors, for adhering to the rules and expectations, and for how they react in trying or frustrating circumstances if you want your teen to be accountable. Everyone in the family should be prohibited from modifying the rules to suit their requirements or sentiments.

Participate in Their Lives

Research repeatedly demonstrates that kids with involved parents are more likely to be responsible and perform better academically, and less likely to engage in dangerous behaviors, including drug use, criminal activity, and sex. Establish open, cordial, and honest contact with your kids from an early age. Discover their hobbies, then participate in their activities. Making your kid feel valued by demonstrating your concern and support can increase their desire to interact with you and do as you ask.

Avoid Getting Too Attached

There is a delicate line between telling your kid that you support them and micromanaging their lives. Many of us do things for our children today as parents that we could and were expected to do for ourselves as kids. Our parents didn't frequently feel the need to bargain with our sports coach, handle every issue we had, or keep us occupied during downtime. Teenagers should be allowed to run their own lives.

Allow for Natural Outcomes

No matter how difficult, you must let your kid take responsibility for their good and bad choices. Although it may seem cruel, it is the best parenting you can do. Teens should pay the fine if they receive a speeding ticket, not you. He must find a means to make money if he still needs to get it, or he risks losing his license. Do not finish a large assignment for your teen if they put it off. Don't forgive your teen's lack of preparation for a test or ask the teacher for a second chance. Let them take the failing grade and deal with the consequences.

Establish Limits

To ensure that your kids understand the repercussions of their conduct, you must set clear and challenging expectations for them. Your teen needs to understand that there will be repercussions if they decide to break the rules. This only works, of course, if you don't give in or give up because your teen complains or makes promises to behave. To witness a change in conduct, you must see the punishment through.

Whenever They Show Responsibility, Compliment Them

Your teen's responsible behavior must be appreciated, motivating them to continue. Never undervalue the impact of praise.

When Are You Ready to Delegate Responsibility to Your Child?

You may need to experiment to determine when and where your child is ready for increased responsibility. Giving your child a genuine say in crucial decisions could begin with using family meetings. This fosters your child's sense of worth. It's a terrific approach to understanding how your youngster makes decisions.

Here are some other factors to think about.

Relative Maturity

Teenagers differ in their maturity levels and propensity to behave responsibly from circumstance to circumstance. Consider their abilities when determining whether your child is prepared for the responsibility. For instance, if a teenager has been responsible while out with friends in the past, their request to visit the city with them can be granted.

Experience

Teenagers must get the chance to resolve specific issues on their own. Experience can also be helpful if there isn't any immediate risk. Your youngster has the chance to demonstrate to you their level of maturity through experience. Additionally, it helps kids develop decision-making skills and confidence.

Legal Aspect

The legal age is the age at which you can legally do things like leave school or your home, obtain a job or a license, agree to sex or for medical treatment, consume alcohol, and other things. Regardless of what other teenagers do or what other parents approve, certain acts must remain on the "no" list until they reach legal age.

Amount of Risk

Teenagers occasionally wish to undertake activities that endanger their safety and wellness because they don't always consider the long-term effects. However, attending a late-night movie showing can be okay if you decide that going to an all-night party carries more risk than reward.

Your Values as a Family

Are you willing to allow your child to make choices or act in a way that goes against your morals? For instance, parents who value kindness and tolerance are likely to prevent their children from acting disrespectfully toward others.

Taking Care of Oneself

Protecting your wants and rights is another reason to set boundaries. If your child asks for something unreasonable or burdens you unfairly, such as spending all day driving kids around or buying expensive equipment, you might say "no."

Giving your child independence in more crucial areas, like going out unattended or making decisions about their studies or future employment, should be your ultimate goal.

What Responsibilities Should You Give Your Teenager?

Teenagers must learn to work independently to mature into responsible adults, but it can be challenging for parents to allow them that opportunity. Sometimes we believe that it will be easier to complete chores on our own, sometimes we don't want to relinquish control, and sometimes we are unsure whether our kids are prepared for new responsibilities. Despite these difficulties, we cannot raise competent adults if we constantly care for their needs. Instead, we must provide them with the tools to care for themselves and contribute to society.

Getting Out of Bed in the Morning

When your child enters middle school, it is time for them to take charge of getting ready for the day. Teenagers can use an alarm clock, get out of bed on time, and get ready for school without aid or reminders. You can help them succeed by showing them how to use the alarm and guiding them through their morning ritual a few times. You can help them adjust to their new responsibilities during the first week. After that, parents should step aside and allow the youngster to work things out independently. There will undoubtedly be instances when your child makes a mistake, such as rushing out the door with only a few minutes to spare, but this does not indicate they are unprepared for this duty. Making mistakes is part of learning, and the repercussions will teach them. If your child misses the bus through no fault of yours, ensure they bear the consequences by informing them ahead of time that they will be obliged to pay you a "taxi" fee for driving them to school.

Making Breakfast and Preparing Their Lunch

Teenagers should prepare their breakfasts and bring their lunches to school. A parent's role is to ensure that their teen's favorite nutritious foods are available in the house so that they may prepare meals. If students fail to complete these responsibilities, they will be hungry or forced to purchase a school meal, which is an excellent motivator to be more responsible in the future. Many parents are concerned that if they relinquish control, their teenagers will eat too little, too much, or in an inconsistent manner. This may be true, but it will happen now when you are still available to provide guidance or after they leave for college and are on their own. Set some restrictions if you are concerned about your teen's eating habits. Create a lunch packing formula for kids to follow, such as one sandwich item, one fruit or vegetable, and one enjoyable snack, such as a sweet or chips. In addition, parents can be in charge of examining lunches before they leave the house.

Completing Assignments or Homework

Current parents are significantly more interested in their children's academics than in earlier generations. While it's wonderful that parents are interested, many cross the line into interference, with some even completing homework for their children. Parents must realize that their child's grades do not reflect their parenting style. The purpose of school is to teach children; if we intervene, our teenagers will not learn anything. Parents may encourage and support their children without doing the work for them or saving them from every academic failure.

Here are some constructive strategies for parents to address their teen's academic difficulties. Keep project materials at home for the procrastinating student. School assignments aren't assigned the night before they're due, so don't rush to the shop for your kid who hasn't planned ahead of time. If they have to stay up late to finish the project, they will experience the side effect of being exhausted. It does not imply that you should rush in to assist. If your teen needs help understanding how to complete a homework assignment, you can encourage them to seek extra assistance from the teacher or hire a tutor. However, you should not finish the work for your teen.

Doing the Laundry

Teens are completely competent in using a washing machine and dryer. Implement this right away, so your college student isn't hauling their laundry home to you every other week. Letting your teen clean their clothes teaches them an independent life skill, lowers your daily workload, keeps teens from getting upset because something important isn't clean when they need it, and provides privacy after nighttime occurrences such as menstrual leaks and wet dreams. It doesn't mean you should never do their laundry, but they should be responsible for the majority of it.

Speaking With Instructors and Coaches

Advocating for oneself is a critical skill for teenagers to learn. If students have a concern with a teacher or coach, they should report the issue to the appropriate authority official. Consider it work-related practice. They must be able to communicate with those in positions of responsibility in their employment; thus, understanding how to articulate their difficulties to those in control is critical to their future. You can undoubtedly assist your kid in determining how to express a concern or what to say, but they must ultimately be the ones who email or speak with the instructor or coach.

Backing off in areas where kids can handle themselves is part of parenting an adolescent. Raising a capable adult requires allowing your kid to attempt new things, face new challenges, experience negative repercussions, negotiate failures, and finally feel confident in themselves.

How Can You Make Your Teenager More Accountable and Responsible?

When moms of teens get together, one of the most common topics is "How to Make Your Teenager Responsible." You know it's possible, don't you? You've seen extraordinarily helpful teenagers or heard of the mythical beast. Is it true that all teenagers are capable of taking on responsibility? Yes, ALL teens are more than capable of taking on the task of modeling responsibility and helpfulness. Let's look at some tips on how to make your teen responsible and teach them to be helpful.

Don't Fix Their Chores

So you say you want your teen to contribute, but what if they don't? Do you rush in to save them? Do you throw your hands up and do it yourself after hours of grumbling and nagging? Worse, do you follow your teen around after they finish a chore to rectify it? Do you wind up redoing the chore because it is so bad? If you have been doing everything for your teenager or following them about "fixing" things, it will take some time (weeks or months) to retrain them (and you) to behave differently).

See What They Are Good at and Assign Chores Accordingly

As previously said, each adolescent is unique. Some teenagers are born leaders. They pick up and assess the situation. If properly trained, these natural leaders will step up and do what is required as situations arise. Other teenagers are more contemplative and cautious by nature. This type will require more structure and clear guidelines to understand what you anticipate from them. It's not that these adolescents are lazy or unwilling to assist. They simply do not want to make a mistake.

Look for the structure and cues your tweens and teenagers require to establish responsible behaviors when working with and teaching them. As you raise your teenagers and tweens, focus on continuous growth rather than whether each child matures similarly.

Model Responsibility Yourself First

Finally, consistent parental modeling can be a significant hurdle in transitioning a seemingly sluggish teen into a motivated teenager! You can't just tell your teen they need to help around the house; you must demonstrate it. Find a happy medium between expecting your teen to assist and modeling the behavior for them. Maintain a consistent schedule and follow through on phone calls and emails to demonstrate accountability. Create daily cleaning routines for your home, make a basic financial plan, and arrive on time to work and school.

Praise Them When They Act Responsibly

Praise your child for their efforts. Take notice of how much work they put in or how efficiently they utilize their time. Make sure they know how grateful you are for their assistance. Or tell them how they saved the day by working for your family. Help them recognize and be proud of how much better your family functioned that day due to all their assistance!

Talk About Consequences and Be Strict About Implementing Them

Now that we've created a solid basis for raising responsible teens, trained our teens, assigned them responsibilities, divided up household chores, and rewarded them, it's time to back it up with penalties! Teach your adolescents responsibility for their actions by making them face the consequences if they do not finish their chores. Natural consequences can be used. They won't have something decent to wear to school or church if they don't keep up with their laundry. You can also assign repercussions. When kids are late getting out the door for school, they must go to bed a half-hour earlier the following night.

Be on the Same Page With Your Partner/Co-Parent

Make it a point in your family to emphasize the importance of being responsible and helpful. To do this, parents in the household must work as a TEAM! This implies that all parental adults in your home must reinforce the same message. If one parent emphasizes the importance of hard work while the other emphasizes that they do not want their children ever to struggle, you have two contradicting messages in your home!!! YIKES! This is not good, and encouraging children to listen and obey will be even more difficult.

Train Them on How the Work Is Done

We may think that our 13- or 14-year-old should know how to care for the house or prepare a meal. After all, they've been on the planet for quite some time, or is it just my perception? Anyway, don't skip this step in training your adolescent. When our boys cleaned the bathroom, I couldn't tell they'd done anything. As I became agitated, I decided to try a different approach. I decided to show them how to clean the bathroom once more. Perhaps I hadn't done it in a while. Perhaps I had stopped assisting them as they grew older, but I had never clearly stated what I expected them to do when I said, "Clean the bathroom." So the next time they cleaned the bathroom, I joined them. I demonstrated exactly what I desired. After that, I stated that I would check them after it was completed and show them what they had missed. It was successful. I wonder if they decided they didn't want mom working with them or if they needed to be shown more carefully. The result was achieved!! So, before you get upset, ensure you've actually trained your children to do the job assigned to them.

Teaching Them Responsibility Is a Lot of Work to Be Prepared For

To raise a responsible adolescent, we must give our adolescent responsibilities! One trap I've noticed is that as a child enters their tween years and complains about work, parents start assigning fewer and fewer household chores. THIS WILL NOT WORK. If a person has fewer responsibilities, they should have plenty of time to complete one or two assignments. Many parents, for example, back off and tell their teenagers that all they want is for them to show up to school and keep their rooms clean. Isn't it simple? When a teenager needs to be given more to do, it usually happens that they have too much time, don't schedule it, and spend it doing stupid, fun things. When the teenager is asked to assist, they panic because they haven't accomplished anything and thus cannot assist you. Assign sufficient household responsibilities to allow them to balance their schoolwork, activities, and job duties. However, ensure they are under natural pressure to work hard and use their time wisely. Help them see that they are more capable than they previously thought!

Don't Be Shy to Use Reinforcements When You Need Them

Most teenagers (and adults) require routines and habits. Most teenagers will pitch in if we always clean up the dishes right after dinner because it is typical and expected. Parenting will be easier if you are consistent! However, we need to be more consistent if the dishes are sometimes left for the following day or are only partially cleaned up. As a result, there will be whining when you tell them to clean the dishes or help you clean them. They want to be free of them. After all, you left them the night before.

Establish Some Basic Routines and Household Expectations

Consider all of the chores that must be completed in the household daily and those that must be completed several times a week and once a week. Divide household responsibilities and assign them to individuals. You can assign the same chore to the same child daily or divide the chores among the children. Create basic household rules next. When all of our kids were home, we had a rule that no dishes were left in the bedrooms and that shoes were to be removed when entering the house. Everyone in our family knew and followed our household rules.

How to Teach Your Kid the Consequences of Their Actions

Children appear to be hardwired to push the boundaries. This can sometimes mean that parents try and try again to get their children to listen to them—and learn to make better choices in the future—but it is often futile. Understandably, parents become discouraged and frustrated when their children refuse to listen and frequently disregard warnings of impending disciplinary measures.

To combat this, have a clear plan when rules are disregarded. Consequences should be used more effectively to reduce misbehavior and teach expectations. The good news is that a few simple adjustments to your discipline methods can significantly impact your children's behavior.

Consequences, when given and enforced correctly, can make your child sit up and take notice that you mean business. However, make an effort to implement them in a firm, kind manner that prioritizes encouraging better behavior over punishment. The goal of using consequences is not to humiliate, embarrass, shame, or make your teen feel unloved. The method should help them understand and remember that misbehavior has negative consequences, such as losing their electronics, that they want to avoid in the future.

Maintain Consistency

Positive and negative consequences are only practical if they are applied consistently. If you take away your children's video games only two out of every three times they hit a sibling, they are unlikely to learn not to do so. Inconsistently imposing consequences sends the message that you aren't serious about what you say and that you can be persuaded to change your mind. As a result, the best approach is to punish children every time they violate a rule. You can also assign positive consequences to actions you want to see more of.

Consistency is essential in teaching children that they cannot get away with bad behavior. Make sure you also stick to the consequences. Don't give in too soon if you take away a privilege for the entire day. Make a firm commitment to doing what you say and saying what you mean. It may take some time for your child to realize and trust that you will follow through, but they will figure it out if you stick with it. Then your children's behavior will likely change—and they will begin to listen to you again!

Focus on the Positive

A healthy, caring relationship with your children is required for discipline. Consequences will be far more effective if your children respect you. So, at the very least, give your children 15 minutes of positive attention daily. The more you invest in quality time with your child, the less time they will spend in time-out. This time could be spent attentively listening to your child while they talk or going for a walk together. You could do a simple baking project, read a favorite story, or bring out old photos and talk about shared memories. The point is that this is their moment. Make an effort to give them your undivided attention. So, no peeking at your phone when you think no one is looking.

Define the Effect Clearly

Consequences should be time-bound. "You're grounded until I say so" isn't specific enough. "You can't go anywhere until I can trust you again," is more effective. Giving consequences with a hazy end date may indicate that you're not serious and are simply making an empty threat in the heat of the moment. Your child may also get the impression that everything will blow over soon. Alternatively, your child may perceive you as being overly strict. If they believe they will never be able to regain your favor, they have little incentive to begin complying.

Always specify how long the penalty will be in effect. Often, 24 hours is a reasonable amount of time to deprive children of something. Try saying, "You've lost your electronics until this time tomorrow.". You may also want to deprive your children of a privilege until they earn it back. In this case, the consequences are designed to encourage positive behaviors such as completing school assignments on time or keeping their bedroom tidy. If this is the case, explain precisely what needs to be done for your children to earn back what has been taken away. This clarifies their expectations and keeps the situation neutral rather than ambiguous or hostile. This method also emphasizes the link between your child's behavior and the outcome. Instead of saying, "You can't have your phone back until I trust you," say, "You can earn your phone back for one hour a night when all of your homework is completed."

Immediate Repercussions

The best outcomes are immediate. Taking away your children's plans overnight with Grandma next week is less effective than taking away their electronics. Immediate consequences help children remember why they got themselves into trouble in the first place. They're more likely to forget what rule they broke If It's delayed by a week. Furthermore, experiencing the consequence immediately following the misbehavior can help motivate them not to repeat it.

However, there may be times when immediate consequences are not possible. The consequences will undoubtedly be delayed if you discover your children were involved in a bus accident three days ago. If they misbehave right before they leave for school in the morning, you may need to wait until they get home before outlining and enforcing a consequence. When it is impossible to make the consequence immediate, inform your children as soon as possible. Make it clear why they're in trouble now by reminding them of the rule they broke.

Use Consequences to Teach

There is a distinction to be made between consequences and punishments. Consequences should be used to teach students. They are not intended to shame children like punishments frequently do. Punishments frequently exacerbate rather than alleviate behavioral issues. Logical consequences, on the other hand, teach better choices by ensuring that the consequence corresponds to the misbehavior. So, if your children refuse to turn off their video games, take them away. Take away the bike if they ride it outside the designated boundaries.

If your older child does not study and fails a school exam, the natural result is a failing grade. A logical consequence can also be imposed, such as losing video game privileges, taking on extra household chores, or missing out on social activities. Give older children and teenagers a say in determining the consequences of various infractions. You may discover that they are even harsher on themselves than you are—and that they are more accepting of the consequences when they have a say in determining what they will be.

Make It Age-Related

Experts agree that effective discipline necessitates a consequence approach that is developmentally appropriate for your children. For example, if a child under the age of three violates a rule, you may choose to remind them that if it happens again, they will receive a time-out. With small children, simply reminding them of the consequences is often enough to influence their behavior. Of course, you must be prepared to take action if they do not comply. If the rule is broken again, remove your child from the situation for a predetermined amount of time (one minute per year of age is a good starting point). Allowing children aged three and up to plan their time-out is an option. "You will need to take a time-out right now, but you can return when you feel ready and in control," you say. This encourages self-management skills and teaches your child self-control. It can also work well with older children and teenagers.

Change It Up

When consequences are used too frequently or for too many things at once, they may lose effectiveness. Children consistently denied privileges for an extended period may lose motivation to earn them back. For example, time-out becomes less effective when used multiple times throughout the day. Or the consequence you are using may not be the best one to elicit the desired changes. Limiting another privilege would be more effective if you usually limit screen time.

Effectively using consequences can make a huge difference in your parenting and your children's behavior. If, despite using these techniques, they still require frequent discipline, consider what else may be contributing to their behavioral issues. Reward systems, praise, and active ignoring are some other positive discipline tools to try. These positive discipline techniques can be highly beneficial in assisting children in making positive changes. A comprehensive approach that includes consequences motivates them to improve their behavior while also helping improve your relationship with them.

Segue: The next chapter will talk about how to talk about puberty and why it is important.

CHAPTER 3: R: RACE AGAINST HORMONES

Humans go through a stage known as adolescence as they grow from children to adults. Adolescence is a period in a person's life when they experience significant social, environmental, and biological changes. The start of puberty, which usually occurs around adolescence, is a critical period in human physical and emotional development. In addition to the visible body changes during this time, the brain of an adolescent undergoes invisible changes. They are controlled by hormones that assist the body in growing taller, changing shape, and even growing hair. Hormones affect various body parts such as bones, muscles, and skin, and the brain produces various essential hormones for puberty. Scientists are learning more about how hormones influence how the brain grows and changes and how this affects how you act and feel.

Why Do Parents Need to Talk About Puberty?

On TV and online, kids see and hear a lot about sex and relationships. They may be familiar with some advanced concepts by the time they reach puberty. However, discussing puberty is still an essential task for parents because not all of this other information is reliable. Don't wait for your children to ask you about their changing bodies. They might not, especially if they are unaware that it is acceptable to question you about this sensitive subject. Talking about puberty is not a one-time event. Discuss with your children the changes their bodies will undergo as they grow. Some girls begin puberty at the age of eight, while some boys begin at the age of nine. As a result, you should begin these discussions early.

The Best Time for Parents to Start Talking About Puberty

Puberty typically begins in girls between the ages of 8 and 14. Before their daughters' periods begin, parents should discuss menstruation with them. Girls can be scared by the sight and location of blood if they don't know what's going on. Most girls have their first period around the age of 12 or 13, about 2 or 2 1/2 years after puberty. However, some people get their periods as early as age 9, while others get them as late as 16. Puberty typically begins in boys between the ages of 9 and 15 years. Boys typically begin puberty later than girls, who usually start around 10 or 11.

Many children receive some sex education in school. Boys and girls are frequently taught separately. Girls are more likely to hear about menstruation and training bras, whereas boys are more likely to hear about erections and changing voices. However, girls should learn about the changes that boys go through, and boys should learn about those that affect girls. Check with teachers about their lesson plans to see where the gaps are. It's a good idea to review the lessons with your child again because children frequently have questions about specific topics.

Changes Parents Should Expect During Puberty

The hormonal changes that occur during puberty cause sexual and other physical maturation. It is difficult to predict when puberty will occur in boys. Some changes occur gradually rather than as one event. Each adolescent male is different the following are the average ages at which puberty changes may occur:

- Puberty onset: 9.5 to 14 years old.

- The first pubertal change is testicular enlargement.

- Penis enlargement begins about a year after the testicles begin to enlarge.

- Pubic hair appears at 13.5 years.

- Fourteen-year-olds have wet dreams.

- Fifteen-year-olds have facial hair, their voice deepens, and they develop acne.

Girls go through puberty the same way as boys, but their puberty usually starts before boys their age. Each girl is unique, and she may experience these changes differently. The following are the average ages at which puberty changes occur:

- Puberty begins between the ages of 8 and 13 years.

- Breast development is the first pubertal change.

- Pubic hair growth occurs shortly after breast development.

- 12-year-olds have hair under their arms.

- Menstrual periods range from 10 to 16.5 years old.

When it comes to secondary sexual characteristics, both boys and girls go through specific stages of development. These are male and female physical characteristics that do not affect reproduction, such as voice changes, the appearance of pubic hair, body shape, and facial hair. The following is a synopsis of the changes that occur.

The first puberty change in boys is the enlargement of the scrotum and testes. The penis does not enlarge at this point. The penis then grows longer as the testes and scrotum grow larger. Following that, the penis will continue to expand in both size and length.

The development of breast buds is the first puberty change in girls. This is the time when the breasts and nipples rise. At this time, the areolas (the dark area of skin that surrounds the breast nipples) expand. The breasts then continue to grow in size. The nipples and areolas will eventually rise again. They then create a new projection on the breasts. Only the nipple remains standing above other breast tissue in adults.

Girls and boys develop pubic hair in the same way. Hair growth begins with long, soft hair that grows only in a small area around the genitals. As the hair grows longer, it becomes darker and coarser. Pubic hair eventually resembles adult hair, albeit in a smaller area. It may spread to the thighs and, on rare occasions, up the stomach.

How to Explain Puberty to Your Kids

When children are toddlers or preschoolers, they begin to inquire about their bodies and yours. It can be stressful if you're not prepared or confident in your answers, but it doesn't have to be! If you start early and talk to them frequently, it will be much easier to talk to them about puberty when they are older. Here is how to explain to teens about their changing bodies as they progress from a young preschooler to an older child experiencing puberty. You and your children will feel more at ease with the correct answers.

How to Open the Conversation

Be reassuring when discussing puberty with children. With so many changes happening at this time, it's easy for kids to feel insecure and alone. Puberty often causes children to be self-conscious about their appearance. It can help them to understand that these changes, many of which are awkward, are common. They should also be aware that the timing of these changes can vary greatly. Acne, mood swings, growth spurts, and hormonal changes are all part of growing up, and everyone goes through them at different rates.

Puberty can begin in girls as early as second or third grade. It can be uncomfortable if your daughter is the first in her friend group to receive a training bra, for example. She may feel isolated and awkward. Changes in boys include the cracking, deepening of the voice, and the growth of facial hair. A boy who is an early or late bloomer may feel awkward or as if he is the target of stares from his peers.

When to Stop

Inform your child that you are available to talk, but also initiate conversations. Discuss puberty and the feelings that accompany it as openly as possible. Parents may feel embarrassed discussing these sensitive topics, but children are often relieved to have them take the lead now and then. It is beneficial to review the material. So, ensure you have your answers before answering your child's questions. If you need help with how to approach the subject of puberty, practice what you're going to say first. Let your child know that while it may be uncomfortable, it is necessary to discuss it. If you have any questions or concerns about puberty and development, consult your child's doctor.

How to Handle Confusion and Depression During Puberty

Your child's emotions are stronger and more intense during puberty. Their mood may shift more quickly, frequently, and erratically. Your child may experience intense emotions that they have never felt before. It is common for them to be perplexed, scared, or angry for no apparent reason. They may also be more sensitive and easily upset than usual. Your child's brain is adjusting to all the new hormones simultaneously with their body. During puberty, the brain begins to strengthen areas that allow them to experience intense and complex emotions. However, the part of the brain responsible for emotional regulation, deep thought, reasoning, and decision-making is frequently the last to develop. Because your child may not yet have the mental capacity to cope with their emotions, they may feel out of control, causing even more irritability and frustration.

Here are some suggestions to assist them in processing and coping with these new emotions:

- Maintain your calm, listen, and acknowledge their emotions.

- Assist them in comprehending their moods and what they may be experiencing.

- Maintain clear rules, boundaries, and expectations.

- Encourage your child to solve problems rather than jumping in to fix them!

- Make the most of "up" times by frequently praising good behavior.

- Collaborate to find ways to lift their spirits and express their emotions.

- Encourage healthy eating and sleeping habits.

- Allow them time to process their emotions and be available when needed.

Explaining How Different Milestones Have a Different Timeline for Everyone.

Puberty begins when the hypothalamus creates gonadotropin-releasing hormone (GnRH). The hypothalamus sends this hormone to the pituitary gland to encourage production of luteinizing hormone (LH) and follicle-stimulating hormone (FSH) by the pituitary gland. The hormones travel to the sex organs (ovaries and testes), stimulating the release of sex hormones (estrogen and testosterone). These messenger hormones initiate the telltale signs of puberty.

When Does Puberty Begin in Boys?

Boys enter puberty between the ages of 9 and 14. Boys reach puberty two years later than girls. However, black and Hispanic boys reach puberty earlier than white boys. If your son begins to show signs of puberty before age nine, consult with his pediatrician about these early changes. Similarly, if no signs of puberty have appeared by age 15, consult with his pediatrician about this delay.

What Are the Puberty Stages for Boys?

For boys, puberty is divided into five stages.

Prepubertal is the first stage. Boys haven't seen any visible changes at this point.

Physical changes begin in Stage 2. Typically, between the ages of 9 and 14, boys begin to experience the following:

- sexual development (growth of their testicles and scrotum)

- sparse hair growth around their penis and under their arms

- height gain (typically 2 to 21/2 inches per year) and possible growing pains

Physical changes accelerate in Stage 3. Between the ages of 10 and 16, boys go through the following:

- continued development of their penis and testicles and the possibility of "wet dreams" (ejaculation during the night while they are sleeping).

- darkening and coarsening pubic hair in their genital area, forming a triangle

- continued increase in height (by about 23/4 to just over 3 inches per year).

- increased sweating, resulting in body odor

- vocal alterations (and cracking in the process)

- an increase in muscle mass

Gynecomastia, or breast development, occurs in approximately 50% of all teenage boys, but it usually resolves by the end of puberty. It is most common in children aged 11 to 15. You should consult your child's healthcare provider if this becomes a physical or social issue.

Puberty reaches a climax in Stage 4. Boys between the ages of 11 and 16 go through the following:

- penis enlargement and darkening of the skin on the scrotum and testicles

- rugae, or red ridges on their testicles, will begin to form

- body hair growth that reaches adult proportions

- the pubic hair remains in a rough triangle

- a peak growth spurt of nearly four inches per year

- acne development

- the voice continued to crack

The final stage is Stage 5. This is the last stage of puberty. Boys complete their physical and mental development. Many people will not develop facial hair until this point in the process. Some boys' pubic hair may extend to their thighs, and others may have a line of hair up to their belly button. Most boys stop growing by 17, but some may continue to grow into their early twenties.

What if Puberty Comes on Too Soon or Too Late?

Everyone is not on the same schedule. Some boys experience early puberty, which is known as precocious puberty. Others may notice changes later, a condition known as delayed puberty.

Early (precocious) puberty: If your son shows signs of puberty before age nine, contact his doctor. This could indicate a pituitary gland or neurological problem. As soon as you suspect a problem, your son's healthcare provider should evaluate him.

Among the possible causes of early puberty are:

- the pituitary gland produces hormones too early

- hypothyroidism, which is an underactive thyroid gland

- a tumor on or near the adrenal gland

If the issue is hormonal, an endocrinologist can prescribe puberty blockers to prevent puberty until the appropriate time comes. Puberty blockers are drugs that prevent your child's body from producing the sex hormones that cause puberty's physical changes. If your son's doctor suspects another problem, he may be referred for additional testing.

Delayed puberty: If your son begins puberty after age 14 or is not progressing through puberty, you should consult with his healthcare provider. Your son may be a late bloomer, especially if his father was as well.

However, hormonal or endocrine abnormalities can also cause puberty to be delayed. If your child's doctor suspects an underlying problem, he will most likely be referred to a specialist for additional testing.

When Do Females Reach Puberty?

Girls typically reach puberty two years earlier than boys. Girls typically enter puberty between the ages of 8 and 13. However, black and Hispanic girls begin puberty younger than white girls (age 7 instead of 8).

What Are the Puberty Stages for Girls?

The Tanner stages also outline the puberty stages for girls and when they are likely to occur. Tanner stages for breasts and pubic hair are distinct. The Tanner stages can be an excellent guide to the changes your daughter will go through. Girls go through five puberty stages.

Prepubertal is the first stage. Girls haven't seen any visible changes at this point.

Physical changes begin in Stage 2. Girls between the ages of 8 and 13 are more likely to notice the following changes:

- Their breasts start to bud, and their areolas (the pigmented area around the nipple) expand.

- There is some pubic hair.

- Height grows by approximately 2.75 inches per year.

Physical changes accelerate in Stage 3. Between the ages of nine and fourteen:
- Their breasts continue to develop.

- Underarm hair begins to grow, followed by pubic hair, which is coarse, curly, and triangle-shaped.

- There is a growth of over 3 inches per year.

- The skin is now more oily, and acne appears.

Puberty reaches a climax in Stage 4. Between the ages of ten and fifteen:
- Their breasts continue to develop, and their nipples begin to protrude.

- The pubic hair remains in a triangle, with far too many hairs to count.

- Growth may continue at a rate of approximately 2 3/4 inches per year.

- Acne problems may persist.

- Periods (menstruation) usually begin around 12 (around the same age as their mothers' and sisters' periods). Some girls, particularly those suffering from disordered eating, begin later.

What if Puberty Comes on Too Soon or Too Late?

Not everyone experiences puberty at the same time. Some girls experience early puberty, which is known as precocious puberty. Some girls don't realize changes until later, a condition known as delayed puberty.

Precocious (early) puberty: A few red flags indicate abnormal female development. Examples include:

- Before their eighth birthday, they begin to show signs of puberty.

- Body changes happen quickly.

- Changes in the body that occur "out of order," such as beginning periods before developing breasts.

- There is a significant gap between when pubic hair appears and breasts develop.

If any of these occur, notify your child's healthcare provider. Simple tests can help determine the cause of precocious puberty.

- The pituitary gland may have "activated" the hormones too soon.

- A tumor may have developed on the adrenal gland.

- Your daughter could have come into contact with estrogen (through estrogen cream, for instance).

Your child's doctor may assess your daughter's progress or send her for specialized tests. An endocrinologist may recommend puberty blockers to delay puberty until the right time comes. These are drugs that inhibit the body's production of sex hormones that cause physical changes during puberty.

Delayed puberty: If your daughter begins puberty late or does not appear to progress through puberty, consult her healthcare provider. She could be a late bloomer if her mother was one. Other possibilities include hormonal imbalances and disordered eating. If your child's doctor suspects an underlying problem, they may refer your child to a specialist for testing and treatment.

Puberty can be an exciting but challenging time in your child's life. Your child may go through many emotional changes in addition to physical changes. Puberty usually begins between the ages of 8 and 14. Contact your child's healthcare provider if you have any concerns about their development. They can assess your child's development and make recommendations.

Things Parents Should Talk About and What Not to Talk About

While you may dislike being reminded of your child's rapidly changing body and emerging sexuality, puberty is a life transition that parents and teens must navigate together. Children are especially vulnerable to depression and engaging in various risky behaviors during puberty. Conversations with your child regularly may help them cope better with these physical and emotional changes.

The following are some dos and don'ts to help you along:

Do Consult Your Neighbors, Friends, and Pediatrician for Advice.

"How did you discuss this with your children?" "What would you do differently?" and "What advice would you give to me?"

Be Open and Honest About Your Feelings About Dating, Sex, and Marriage.

Teens who had more sexual health conversations with their parents than their friends were more likely to believe that sex should wait until marriage (DiClemente et al., 2001).

Take Advantage of the Internet's Power

A simple Google search for "How do I talk to my child about puberty?" will yield helpful books, articles, websites, and parenting blogs. Boston Children's Hospital, Kids Health, and the American Academy of Pediatrics have some useful websites.

Refrain From Cramming Everything Into a Single Conversation

You might recall "the talk" with your parents. However, having frequent, smaller conversations can be more effective when it comes to your children. Use everyday experiences to bring up the subject. For example, you've probably seen an embarrassing love scene while watching a movie or TV show with your child. You either ignored what happened or changed the channel awkwardly. Instead, use this as an opportunity to learn what your child thinks and to express your thoughts on this behavior.

Don't Take Notice of the Eye-Rolling or Exaggerated Sighing

Their eyes may be turned away from you, but their ears remain open! Although your children may be embarrassed, studies show they still want to learn from you. Ask your child what they already know about puberty as a starting point.

Don't Underestimate the Power You Have Over Your Child's Behavior

In one study, parent-child sexual health communication was linked to decreased sexual activity and increased confidence in refusing sex. Teens who had sex were more likely to use condoms and other contraception.

Don't Assume Your Children "Know Everything" About Puberty and Sex

Yes, teens learn about puberty and sex from movies, television, music videos, and peers, but none of these sources are as good as you. Most states (including Pennsylvania) do not mandate sex education in schools. Even if they do, you can't be sure they're teaching what you want them to. Your school district's health education experiences will vary greatly. This information is frequently available on the website of your school district.

Segue: The next chapter will talk about sex, the hard, sensitive talk.

CHAPTER 4: E: ENGAGING CONVERSATIONS

Dear parents, have you tried having the birds and bees talk? Do you just turn around whenever you're about to have a talk with them, failing to find the right words? Well...let's see if this helps you.

Why Should Parents Talk About Sex?

Curiosity about sex develops naturally as a result of learning about the body. Sex education teaches children about the human body and helps them feel good about themselves. Younger children are more interested in pregnancy and babies than in the mechanics of sex.

Discussing sex is also essential to establishing open communication with your child. Early, honest, and open communication between parents and children is critical, especially as your child approaches adolescence. If open communication is regular, children are likely to talk to their parents about other challenges of adolescence, such as anxiety, relationships, depression, drug and alcohol use, and sexual issues.

The best sex education strategy is to start a conversation about sex early and keep it going as the child grows. It allows parents to avoid having a long and possibly uncomfortable conversation with their children when they reach adolescence. They're likely to have gotten the information or misinformation about it from their friends. These conversations are easiest to have when prompted by a life experience, such as seeing a pregnant woman or a baby.

When parents discuss sex with their children, they can ensure that they receive accurate information. Parents should be a child's first source of sex information. Understanding correct information can keep children safe as they grow older.

Promoting Family Values

Sex education also allows you to instill your family values in your children. If the subject has never been discussed before, there is a good chance that your adolescent will reject this message. If parents do not teach their children about sex, they will find out about it elsewhere. A teen's exposure to sex information starts earlier than most parents believe. If parents do not discuss sex with their children, they will have little control over what and how their children learn about sex.

School, Playground, and the Media

Parents should not rely on the school system to teach their children about sexuality. Sex education may or may not be available where you live. If your child is receiving sex education at school, go over it with them. Inquire about what they discovered. What a child learns in school, from friends, and on social media is likely to be incomplete and incorrect. It could also be humiliating or even dangerous.

Although there is a lot of sex and sexuality in the media, it is often portrayed sensationally and superficially. Realistic depictions of relationships and sexuality are uncommon. More often than not, sex and sexuality issues appear in isolation, without any emotional or relationship context. Furthermore, the dangers of sexual activity are frequently exaggerated in the media.

Sex Education Is Preferable to No Sex Education

According to studies, the more children are exposed to sexual images in the media, the more likely they are to engage in sexual behavior at a young age. Basic sex education, on the other hand, does NOT result in promiscuity. Children exposed to sex education at home are less likely to engage in risky sexual behavior.

Open communication about sex and other topics with children is both healthy and safer in the long run. This does not imply that it will be simple or without awkward moments. Teenagers are still very private individuals. However, discussing sex early increases teens' likelihood of approaching parents when difficult or dangerous situations arise.

How to Talk to Your Kids About Sex

It is not always easy to parent a teen. Youths require adults to connect, communicate, spend time with them, and demonstrate genuine interest in them. Talking with teens about sex-related topics, such as healthy relationships and the prevention of HIV, other sexually transmitted diseases (STDs), and pregnancy, is a well-researched positive parenting practice. Various programs have been shown to increase the amount and quality of communication between parents and their teens in various settings (e.g., schools and parents' workplaces).

What Can Parents Do

When parents communicate with their adolescent child about sex, relationships, HIV, STDs, and pregnancy prevention, they promote their child's health and lessen the likelihood of them engaging in risky behaviors. The following are some actions and approaches parents can take to improve communication with their teens about these difficult-to-discuss health issues.

Understand Where Your Teen Obtains Information

What health messages is your adolescent receiving? What health messages are true and medically correct? Teachers, health care providers, friends, television, or social media may send your teen messages about sex, relationships, and the prevention of HIV, STDs, and pregnancy. Some messages contain incorrect information. Avoid assuming that health education class covers everything you want the teen to know. Remember, school curricula vary by state.

Begin Talking as Soon as Possible and Keep the Conversation Going

We must start talking to our children as soon as possible and keep the conversation going. Even young children must learn about self-respect, appropriate touch, and consideration for the feelings and limits of others. When these topics feel like an essential part of the values you regularly discuss, they will be much easier to discuss as your children enter puberty and develop sexual feelings.

In general, teens find it easier to talk about values and safety as an ongoing conversation rather than as a reaction to an event. In other words, if your conversation does not begin before a first date or prom night, you will be much more at ease—and your adolescent will be much more receptive. Ongoing conversations have the feel of education and can be treasured as opportunities to clarify values and consider how to make decisions. Conversations held emergently appear to originate from fear and seem controlling or demanding. As a result, even the best intentions can backfire.

Make It About Your Values

Various resources are available for your tween or teen to learn about the mechanics of sex or the details of puberty and development. Health classes, books, and the internet are examples. You must ensure that they learn the values associated with healthy sexuality from you. If you and other caring adults do not address these issues, your children will learn their values from the internet, television, and music. In the worst-case scenario, they will be exposed to harmful and disturbing depictions of sex and sexuality through internet pornography. They'll also learn from their peers, and while those values may be sound, they won't be seasoned by life experience.

Listen

Pay attention to what your tweens and teens say about sexuality. The more they confide in us, the better we will be able to guide them toward developmentally appropriate sex solutions. Listening to our teenagers is essential for getting them to talk to us. Sometimes fewer words from us mean more words from them.

Encourage them to speak up. When they ask a question, inquire about what they already know or have heard about the subject. Take a nonjudgmental listening stance. Be truthful in your responses to them as well. Take note of how people react to your responses. If you cannot answer a question immediately, say you will work to obtain the necessary information and follow up with them later.

Create Teachable Moments Using Social Media

Nowadays, there is a lot of sexuality in the media. While this may bother us, we can benefit from it. Television shows, movies, websites, books, and magazines can all be used to teach young people about sexuality. Our teenagers may be more likely to ask or answer questions because the "storylines" are about people other than themselves. That's because they're listening in on conversations about people they don't know.

Make Sexuality Appear a Beautiful Aspect of Being Human

Too often, when discussing sex with our tweens and teens, we only discuss the dangers and consequences of sexual behavior. But what about all the positive aspects and emotions associated with sexuality? Do you recall feeling butterflies in your stomach after your first "crush?" What about the joy you felt when you discovered that someone you liked actually liked you back? Or the rush of joy after your first kiss? Our teens need to hear about the joys of sexuality from us as caring adults. We must teach them to appreciate the bodies they have been given to ensure that they understand what their bodies are capable of and how to keep them healthy. You can discuss with your child the safety and emotional benefits of abstinence while discussing the usual feelings that come with developing sexual awareness.

Get a Trusted Professional

You are not by yourself. Your role as a parent is critical, and you are un-questionably a valued and trusted advisor to your adolescent. However, the most effective parents collaborate with other trusted adults to create a multi-layered blanket of protection for their children. Even in the most comfortable and openly communicating families, adolescents will seek guidance from other adults. Sex and sexuality, in particular, are topics on which young people want privacy while also seeking guidance. Parents are indispensable when it comes to discussing values and mutual respect, whereas professionals may be more comfortable offering specific messages about self-protection.

Teens say their parents, not friends, have the most influence over their sexual decisions, but only if their parents talk to them. As difficult as it seems, open and honest talk about sexuality shapes our teens into better-prepared adults for healthy, meaningful relationships.

Why Should Parents Talk About Sexuality?

Your kids should be able to tell you how they feel about their sexuality, and this doesn't happen until you initiate the conversation. You must be open to new questions and ideas. If the questions are about homosexuality, your child is not necessarily a homosexual. Perhaps they are simply interested in what happens. Don't draw any conclusions. But it is your initiative that makes all the difference.

How to Talk About Sexuality

Parents may also postpone conversations about sex because they are afraid of implanting ideas in their child's mind before they are "ready" or because they associate talking about sexuality with implicit permission to engage in sexual behaviors. Sex education and parent-child sexuality communication are linked to delayed sexual activity and more consistent contraceptive use. Two to four conversations with parents have the potential to serve as a barometer against which teens measure other information about sexuality and limit early sexual activity.

Parents usually avoid positive topics about sexuality, including pleasure, love, or healthy relationships, for negative topics and warnings. Topics such as sexuality, STDs, pregnancy, abuse, and exploitation are usually missing during these discussions. Adolescents need parental guidance to develop, but they must receive accurate information from medically accurate sources.

Understand It Yourself, Too

The foundation for sexual communication is laid in early childhood. It occurs throughout many interactions and "teachable moments"—opportunities that arise to start a conversation or provide information about a topic—rather than one "big talk" about "the birds and the bees." Regular and ongoing discussions support and reinforce concepts addressed in previous conversations, increasing the likelihood that the content will be encoded to memory and cognitively accessible later. Some parents and adolescents may have discussed sexuality in the past, but not recently. An absence of conversation may indicate that parents should check in with their teens.

Regarding sexuality conversations, parents and children may have different ideas about what constitutes a "conversation." Parents report more frequent sex communication than their teenagers, possibly because they consider a broader range of topics to be sex-related than teenagers, including generalized warnings indirectly related to sex, such as "Stay away from boys. Period." Some parents may rely on such broad statements because they are unsure where to begin or how to be more specific.

Sexual Orientation

Families are diverse, and each child's family is unique. It is most recently not uncommon for someone to have two mothers or fathers. If your children are curious, as most are, they may inquire about it. These questions provide an excellent opportunity to educate your child on essential topics such as sexual orientation and healthy relationships. I've learned communication tips from providing health care to teenagers for the past decade, and I hope they can help you. Let's begin with the fundamentals of sexual orientation.

Explaining Sexual Orientation

"When you think about who you are romantically or physically interested in, who do you picture?" is how I typically explain sexual orientation. "Men, women, both, or neither?" Sexual orientation is both a physical and a romantic attraction. It differs from gender identity. Gender identity refers to how a person perceives themselves on the gender spectrum (such as female, male, or non-binary). Sexual orientation refers to who you believe you are attracted to or who you could see yourself loving.

A lesbian is a woman who is only attracted to women. A gay is a man who is only attracted to men. A bisexual person is attracted to both the male and female genders. A heterosexual is a person who is attracted to the opposite gender. A pansexual is a person attracted to another person without regard for gender. LGBTQ is frequently used to group sexual orientation and gender identity (lesbian, gay, bisexual, transgender, queer, questioning). These are the reality of our world today, and it will be good for parents to understand and then explain to the kids.

Why Should You Talk About It?

According to research, family support is essential. Sexual minority youth (those who identify as lesbian, gay, bisexual, or transgender-LGBTQ) are nearly five times more likely to attempt suicide than their heterosexual peers. Furthermore, LGBTQ youth from highly rejecting families are more than eight times more likely to attempt suicide than their LGBTQ peers from low or no-rejection families. Sexual and gender minority youth are overrepresented in the homeless population (more LGBTQ youth than "straight" youth). The good news is that evidence suggests that parental communication and monitoring can help prevent these adverse outcomes. We can grow as parents and as people with some help to become the people our children require.

How to Talk About Sexual Orientation with Your Teen

Here are some handy tips on talking about sexual orientation with your kids.

Look For Teachable Moments

Teachable moments are everywhere. We have everything from song lyrics to television to meeting people in our community. There are endless opportunities to initiate a conversation with your children. Because it is not intimidating, these moments can relieve stress in both children and parents. "What do you think about that?" is an excellent place to start. Then the next step in the conversation can begin.

Tell Them You Adore Them

Knowing what isn't said is sometimes just as important as knowing what is. For example, two men kiss on TV, and Uncle Joe becomes enraged or makes a crude joke about it. If you never bring it up again, the child may learn that your family disagrees. So, ask your child later how Uncle Joe reacted. For example, "What did you think about Uncle Joe's words while he was watching TV?"

Starting a conversation about it can open the door to further discussion. You can then say, "Can I tell you what I think about it?" You can use that opportunity to share your values and beliefs, even if it is as simple as "I believe people should be free to find the partner they love and trust." To return to the theme of healthy relationships, you could reframe the conversation to ask if they were in love, kissing, or touching on their first date, for example. Then talk about love, its feeling and look, and dealing with physical intimacy when interested in someone, such as kissing, touching, and sex. This is another chance to express your values and beliefs.

It's critical to follow up with your child and let them know they have a safe place to express themselves. We frequently assume that our children understand that we love them no matter what, but this is not always the case. It's good to practice telling them you love them for who they are and that they can talk to you. Choose a trusted adult to whom you can refer them when not comfortable or not willing to talk.

Recognize That Each Child Is Unique

"We have two children, and they frequently hear things in different ways. When I explain things to my now-eight-year-old, he always needs a deep dive, whereas my five-year-old is content with more straightforward explanations," a mother once said. If possible, separate conversations about sexual orientation should be held for those deep dives. Each child has their own set of questions, understandings, and experiences.

Recognize That Pausing Is Acceptable

As a parent, I understand that we may not always be in the right frame of mind for these essential conversations. For example, when driving in rush hour traffic. One piece of advice I can give is that it's okay to return to the conversation. Tell your child that it's an important topic and that you appreciate them bringing it up, and then ask if we can talk about it another time, perhaps when we have a few minutes alone. That is precisely what I did. I might reread some trusted online resources, take a few deep breaths, and then return feeling mentally prepared. If you choose this route, remember to follow up with your child! If I forget, I sometimes ask my child to remind me, and they always seem to remember.

How to Respond to Their Orientation

Your adolescent may have suspected for some time that they are not straight or cisgender and may have struggled to "come out" to you. Even if they feared your reaction, they were brave and honest in telling you about their sexuality or gender identity. The first thing to remember is that their coming out isn't about you or anything you've done. Parenting your child in a certain way does not automatically make them LGBTQ. Whatever your personal feelings about the situation, you must listen to what they say and thank them for confiding in you. Reaffirm that your feelings for them have not changed. If you feel unprepared, upset, or concerned about your LGBTQ child, you can ask them for some time to process what they have told you. You can then use that time to pray, and seek advice or assistance.

Talking Contraceptives with Teens

The first rule is to be forthright and honest with your children about birth control. That means not brushing aside direct questions or crafting flowery responses that sidestep the issue, like talking about the "birds and the bees." It's true regardless of your child's age. Testing your child in a mature manner during its discussion using real terms and straightforward language is a good idea. Children can see through euphemisms and need to know what things are called. You may notice "ewws," weird looks, or feigned disinterest in bringing up the subject. These are normal reactions. So don't be discouraged.

Have the conversation and acknowledge if your child appears disgusted or uninterested. Let them express their emotions and inform them that you believe the information is essential. Even if a child appears to be not listening, they usually are. Sometimes, a child feels overwhelmed, and you can tell they are done. In those cases, put the conversation on hold and pick it up again soon.

In the end, each child and family is unique. As a parent, you are the best person to understand your child's needs and feelings regarding birth control and sex conversations. Some children, for example, benefit from sit-down meals at the dinner table, where they can concentrate. That type of environment may cause anxiety in other children. Some of the best conversations I've heard between parents and children take place in the car or on a walk. What matters is that you have the conversation, not when or where you have it.

Most Common Types of Birth Control

When discussing birth control with your child, it's helpful to have a general understanding of the main types, how they work, and which ones might be best for your child. A teen can use birth control for treating secondary issues, such as severe cramping, irregular periods, or acne. Knowing the following is essential.

Condoms

Condoms are most likely the most easily accessible form of birth control for you. They can be purchased online or in a supermarket. In addition, unlike most forms of contraception, it does not require a prescription. Unless you are allergic to latex or the lubricant commonly found in condoms, the side effects are usually minor. One significant advantage of using condoms is that they can reduce your risk of contracting an STD.

They can also be used with other birth control methods, such as an IUD and the pill, to reduce your chances of becoming pregnant. However, for condoms to be effective, they must be used correctly and consistently, which is not always as simple as it appears.

Implants and IUDs

The implant and IUD are the most effective methods. These are long-term birth control methods, but they can be removed early if desired. You can have them inserted, and forgetting about them is a huge benefit. Compared to the pill, which is taken daily, these options are relatively low maintenance.

The implant is a plastic rod the size of a matchstick inserted beneath your skin. It causes ovulation by releasing the hormone progestin. According to Planned Parenthood, the implant is more than 99% effective. A pelvic exam is not required to obtain an implant, but you must see a healthcare professional to insert it. A pelvic exam and a prescription for IUD insertion are required.

There are two types of IUDs: copper IUDs and hormonal IUDs. The copper IUD is a non-hormonal method, which is advantageous for those who do not wish to use hormonal contraception. Because copper repels sperm, it is effective. Copper IUDs can be left in place for up to 12 years.

The hormonal IUD is worn for three to seven years. It secretes progestin, which inhibits ovulation. Some people find that the hormonal IUD stops or lightens their period. Some people report that implants or IUDs cause painful periods and bad PMS. Unfortunately, predicting how your body will react to these birth control methods is difficult.

Pills for Contraception

Oral contraceptive pills are a popular method of birth control. You can take the mini pill (only progestin) or the combination pill (progestin and estrogen). There are some potential disadvantages. To begin, you must take them at the same time every day for them to be effective. Second, some people experience side effects such as acne or breast tenderness, while others experience unexpected benefits such as lighter periods, less acne, and a more stable mood.

Talking about sexual reproduction, pregnancy prevention, intercourse, and male and female anatomy can be awkward. Your child will always feel like they are your baby, no matter their age. Lean into the awkwardness, push through it, and have these meaningful conversations with your kids. The more accurate information they receive from you and the more informed they are on the subject, the better they will be able to make responsible, safe decisions as they grow older.

Importance of Consent

Consent is when a person is actively involved in a sexual experience and freely agrees to what is going on without being threatened, pressed, intoxicated, or too young. Yes, we realize this is an awkward topic, but it is also essential. Talking about sex and consent with your adolescent teaches them about their rights and what constitutes safe and healthy sex. If you're looking for communication tips, we spoke to some parents about what works for them when discussing general consent and sex.

Here are some suggestions for teaching your teen about consent:

Talk About What Consent Means to Them

Don't assume your adolescent knows or doesn't know what consent entails; instead, use this opportunity to ask them. This will give you an idea of what you need to discuss and any misunderstanding or harmful understanding of consent they may have. Consent must be clear, i.e., only a 'yes' means 'yes,' and any sexual activity without consent is considered sexual assault. Sexual consent is a conversation as someone may decide to stop having sex, even if they have already begun. If this occurs, their partner must respect them and stop immediately.

Discuss How Their Lives Are Changing

When your adolescent is growing up and going through puberty, it can be challenging to think clearly. Assure your teen that these new, potentially overwhelming feelings are normal and that they can always talk to you about them. Help them understand that they must still respect themselves and others regardless of their feelings.

Allow Them To Establish Their Boundaries While Respecting Others

The goal is to give your teen the tools they need to figure out what they're comfortable with and to feel confident communicating those boundaries to their partner in the future. You can help by doing the following:

Encourage them to ask themselves questions like, *Why do I want sex? Do I feel obligated to have sex? Do I feel secure? Is it possible that I'm more nervous than excited?* These aren't questions they need to answer; they're just good prompts to consider when deciding whether or not they're ready for sex.

Remind them that they owe no one sex. It makes no difference if they are in a romantic relationship with another person or are already comfortable kissing or touching their partner. It makes no difference if they've previously had sex. It's also important to understand that saying "I love you" or giving gifts does not obligate them to have sex or do anything in return.

Tell them that it is essential to discuss sex and intimacy with any partner. They should be able to express what they want and don't want to do and how that changes throughout a relationship or interaction.

Discuss the impact they believe their actions will have on others. If you notice your teen objectifying others, remind them that those people are human beings, not just sexual objects. Remind them that consent and respect are two-way streets and that they must also respect the boundaries of their sexual partners.

Encourage Them to Think About What They Understand

Ask them, "How do you know if someone wants to kiss you?" and "How do you know if someone is interested in you?" "How can you tell if your partner is sexually ready?" If you don't think they'll feel comfortable answering such questions in person, you could send them an email or text or ask them to write their answers down on paper. You could also arrange for them to speak with another trusted adult with whom they are comfortable.

Inquire About Their Partying, Drinking, and Drugs

Ask your teen how they plan to protect themselves and their friends while partying. Alcohol and drugs impair someone's ability to consent; if they or someone else is highly drunk or high, they cannot consent. Sexual assault occurs when you engage in sexual activity with someone who cannot give informed consent. Be careful with your language here, and make it clear that the survivor is never to blame for the sexual assault. The perpetrator is always responsible for making the right decision and not harming anyone.

Keep the Conversation Going

Continue discussing consent, respect, and healthy boundaries as your adolescent enters into relationships. Regular discussion normalizes the topic, and your teen will enjoy healthy and respectful relationships. Tell them to always talk to you if they feel their boundaries are violated. Assure them that you will not hold it against them if someone hurts or violates them. You understand that sexual assault is only the perpetrator's fault, regardless of whether they were in the wrong place or had been drinking alcohol. It's also a good idea to talk to your teen about other trusted adults they can talk to if they don't feel comfortable talking to you. Ask your teen, "If something happens and you can't talk to me, who are three people you can talk to?"

Teen Pregnancies

Adolescent pregnancy is a huge problem. When girls are denied the right to make decisions about their sexual and reproductive health and well-being, teen pregnancy rates rise. Girls must be able to make their own decisions about their bodies and futures, understand the consequences of adolescent pregnancy, and have access to appropriate healthcare and sex education.

How Can I Assist My Sexually Active Adolescent in Avoiding Pregnancy?

Discussing the delay in having sex, birth control options such as condoms, and their plans can help teens avoid pregnancy until they are ready. Having life goals and considering how pregnancy might interfere with those goals is an essential step for teens to postpone pregnancy until they are ready.

The most effective way to avoid pregnancy (and STDs) is to use birth control and condoms every time you have sex. Various birth control methods are both safe and effective for teenagers. Discussing birth control, assisting them in obtaining birth control from a trusted doctor, obtaining condoms from a local drugstore, and assisting them in obtaining the facts when it comes to their birth control questions are the best ways to help your teen avoid pregnancy.

Do you suspect your adolescent is sexually active but haven't talked about it? Begin the conversation. Find some alone time with just the two of you. Begin by reminding them that you love them unconditionally and want to talk to them because you care. Inquire whether they are having sex and, if so, whether they are using birth control and condoms. Inform them that you are available to answer any questions they may have.

Talking to an Adolescent About Pregnancy Options, Including Abortion

The first and most important thing you can do is tell them that you love them regardless of what happens and that they can always come to you if they need help deciding which pregnancy option is best for them or if they need help getting an abortion or prenatal care. Even if you believe they will come to you because you are supportive, it is still important to express to them that you would assist them if they became pregnant. Many teenagers are afraid to discuss these issues with their parents for fear of being reprimanded or disappointed. So, reminding them regularly that you love them no matter what and would assist them if they were pregnant can make them feel more at ease and even improve your overall relationship.

You can also discuss with them how deciding what to do about a pregnancy is a very personal decision that should be made by the pregnant person. You discuss values regarding things like people controlling their bodies, a concept known as "bodily autonomy," and empathizing with other people's lives and situations.

Segue: The next chapter will talk about nutrition, and healthy habits.

CHAPTER 5: N: NUANCES OF NUTRITION

Are you tired of seeing your teenager prefer junk food over the nutritious food that you get for them? Do you feel like they should know more about nutrition? What can you do to make them more excited about eating healthy food? Do they sleep well? Are they active and exercising?

How Can You Help Teens to Develop Healthy Eating Habits?

Let's face it: our teenagers have a lot on their plates. They have school or homework, active social lives, extracurricular activities, or part-time jobs. They struggle with healthy eating habits as parents do, regardless of all the pressures. However, good nutrition is essential for adolescents who are going through a lot of changes, and it helps them perform at their best—academically, physically, and emotionally.

Make It as Simple, Straightforward, and Realistic as Possible.

People's eating habits are heavily influenced by convenience. A busy schedule is one of the barriers to healthy eating for teenagers. Stock up on quick but healthy foods and keep them easily accessible. Because we are more likely to try what we see, store healthy snacks in clear containers. Keeping things simple increases the likelihood and sustainability of healthy eating—not just for your teens but also for you.

Keep In Mind That Tastes Change.

When assisting your teen in eating healthier, remember that their tastes and interests will change as they grow older. Tweens eat whatever you serve them, whereas older teens may have new dietary preferences, such as veganism or vegetarianism. Availability of healthy food that fits their new choices will help ensure that they rely on something other than potato chips or cookies because those are the only vegan items in the house.

Examine Your Situation, Needs, and Capabilities.

Making small, long-term changes is the key to eating healthier. Healthy food doesn't have to be expensive. Meal preparation once a week, or even once or twice a month, can save time. Certain foods and cooking methods are part of a family or cultural tradition in many households. In these cases, it is okay to not alter your cooking and eating habits completely, but rather to make small changes that honor tradition while making your meals healthier. For example, you could use low-sodium soy sauce instead of regular soy sauce.

Start Early and Model Healthy Eating.

Keep in mind that our positive eating habits can have a significant impact on our children. Our children are more likely to get their recommended daily servings of fruits and vegetables if we do. Similarly, eating habits are formed early in childhood and can last well into adolescence and adulthood. The earlier you help your children develop healthy eating habits, the more likely they will be to stick with them and turn them into long-term habits. However, there is always time to begin eating healthier, so don't be disheartened if you didn't do enough when your children were younger.

Encouragement

The advantages of eating healthy are their reward. As parents, the best we can do is provide healthy options for our children and offer encouragement and positive reinforcement for making good decisions. Because they are developing their identities and desire independence at this age, they may not always make the best choices when reaching for a snack or grabbing a quick meal with friends. However, by modeling good habits and increasing their awareness of a healthy diet, you ensure that they make informed nutritional choices. So, when you pat your teen on the back for eating healthy, remember to give yourself one.

Sleep and Teenagers

According to sleep research, a teenager requires between eight and ten hours of sleep per night. This is more than a child or an adult requires. Despite this, most adolescents only get 6.5 to 7.5 hours of sleep per night, with some getting less. Chronic sleep deprivation results from not getting enough sleep regularly. This can significantly impact a teenager's life, negatively impacting their mental health and increasing their risk of depression, anxiety, and low self-esteem. It can also have an impact on academic performance at school.

How Much Sleep Is Enough?

Teens enjoy labeling themselves as "night owls," sharing stories of all-nighters and sleeping the entire Saturday away. Though teenagers and their sleeping habits can aggravate parents, they are partly caused by physical changes during puberty. "Teens experience a natural shift in circadian rhythm," says Laura Sterni, M.D., a sleep expert at Johns Hopkins. This makes falling asleep before 11 p.m. more difficult. Add in early school start times, more homework, extracurricular activities, and possibly a part-time job, and sleep deprivation in teens become common. Sterni, on the other hand, believes that parents must assist teens in doing their best because this age group requires more sleep than we may realize.

How Can You Help Teens Get More Sleep?

Many parents begin by asking their adolescent children about their sleep, as surveys show many parents are unaware that their children have sleeping problems. Parents can encourage their children to see a doctor while also working with them to improve their sleep hygiene gradually. According to some studies, teens with a strict bedtime set by their parents get more sleep and have less daytime drowsiness.

Another option for parents is to lobby their local school district for later start times. Several districts have tried delayed starts and found positive attendance and academic performance results. Parents can also work with their teenagers to avoid overscheduling and commitments that can cause stress and interfere with adequate sleep time.

Exercising and You

Teens must exercise to stay healthy. Encouraging healthy lifestyles in children and teenagers is critical for their future success. Childhood lifestyle choices are more likely to be carried over into adulthood. Some lifestyle changes may be more challenging to implement as a person ages. The best way to promote healthy lifestyles is to involve the entire family.

According to physical activity guidelines, teens should engage in one hour or more of moderate to vigorous physical activity per day. The majority of physical activity should be aerobic, involving the use of large muscles over a long period. Running, swimming, and dancing are all examples of aerobic activity. Any moderate to vigorous activity contributes to the 60-minute goal. Muscle- and bone-strengthening physical activity should be included at least three times per week.

Sports and structured exercise programs that include muscle and bone-strengthening activities are appropriate for teenagers. Under the supervision of a qualified adult, weight training can improve strength and help prevent sports injuries. Teens can benefit from activities they enjoy if they have the opportunity and interest, such as skateboarding, yoga, swimming, or dancing. Teens can make physical activity part of their daily lives by doing chores, walking to school, or finding a part-time job.

Motivating Teens to Be Physically Active

According to their parents, teens should control how they choose to be physically active. Give teens the option to make their own decisions. It is not what they do but rather that they are active. Many teens enjoy the well-being, reduced stress, and increased strength and energy that exercise provides once they get started. As a result, some children begin to exercise regularly without prompting from their parents.

Teens need to have fun to stay motivated. Provide equipment, transportation, and companionship for your teen's choices. Peers can impact teenagers' lives, so provide opportunities for them to be active with their peers. Find an exercise plan that works with your teen's schedule to help them stay active. Your teen can participate in a sport at school. However, many gyms have teen memberships, and kids can visit before or after school.

Other teenagers prefer doing home exercise videos, tennis, or bowling. These can be good options, but engaging in moderate to vigorous activities is essential daily. Furthermore, all teenagers should limit their time spent engaging in sedentary activities such as watching TV, playing video games, and using computers, smartphones, or tablets.

Segue: The next chapter will talk about personal hygiene.

Chapter 6: T: Teaching a Teen Hygiene

With their sweat glands more active than before, their body covered with a smattering of coarse hair everywhere, girls starting their menstrual cycle, and boys exploring aspects of their sexuality, teenagers need repeated reminders of hygiene from you. They also need to know how to take care of themselves.

How to Teach Your Kids to Have Good Hygiene

Teaching teens about good hygiene is usually a combination of teaching and gentle reminders. While you've most likely taught them many skills since their childhood, some of these hygiene tasks are new to them or must be completed independently for the first time. It's also common for kids to become less conscientious about personal hygiene as they enter middle and high school, especially when they're no longer groomed under the supervision of their parents. Here's a primer on which healthy hygiene habits to teach your teen and how to incorporate them into their daily routine.

General Hygiene

Hygiene is the process by which we keep our bodies clean. Cleanliness practices serve two primary purposes. To begin with, being clean helps us be sanitary—not wholly free of germs, but mostly harmful germs that can cause disease. Poor hygiene can result in tooth decay, skin infections, and other avoidable illnesses. Second, hygiene has an impact on social interactions. Other people, especially adults, expect people to be clean. Good hygiene enables us to interact more positively with others. Being close to someone with bad breath or body odor can be unpleasant. Proper hygiene shows that you care about and value yourself. It's also courteous to others to present yourself neatly. In contrast, poor hygiene can lead to social rejection.

For Boys

Hygiene refers to how we keep our bodies clean daily. This has two effects. It helps us to be free of germs, if not all of them, then at least the majority of them, and it also helps us to improve our social interaction with other people. Having good hygiene indicates that you take care of yourself.

Showering Every Day

This may sound a little gross, but in many households, boys were the ones who needed to be reminded about showering regularly. Boys have a habit of not caring much, and they can go weeks without it by surviving primarily on other people's scents or deodorants. It's dangerous for the body as the accumulated sweat or dust encourages infections in different body parts. As a result, ensure that your teen takes a shower regularly and does not skip it too often.

Washing the Face

Acne on the face is one of almost every teen's worst nightmares. This is one of the most common teen problems. The main reason for this is a lack of skin care during adolescence. Teen boys are especially vulnerable to this issue because they rarely care for their faces. Teenagers must learn how to wash their face regularly using face wash or cleanser.

Ensure that they do so regularly. Teens must remember to be gentle with their skin and massage their face gently when using a specific face wash or cleanser. Furthermore, people must teach teenagers to massage their faces while applying moisturizers. This aids in the absorption of the cream or lotion by your skin.

Using Deodorant

During the adolescent years, boys participate in various activities, each of which requires a lot of body movement and can result in physical exertion. As a result, the body produces a lot of sweat, which must be cleaned to ensure that it does not cause any infection or anything else. This adolescent needs to shower more frequently. In addition, they must learn to use deodorant or antiperspirant to control their sweating. However, excessive use of antiperspirants may result in sweat gland blockage.

Dental Hygiene

It is undeniable that teens are careless when it comes to maintaining their dental hygiene. Teen boys must brush at least twice daily, floss regularly, and occasionally use mouthwash. This will help prevent or slow the growth of harmful bacteria, which will aid in preventing diseases such as cavities and gingivitis. Self-hygiene will be emphasized if the teen ever takes a personality development course.

Clothes and Shaving

Teen boys have a terrible habit of not changing their clothes regularly, instead wearing the same t-shirt repeatedly. This habit must be broken. Furthermore, hair growth can be seen in various parts of the body during the adolescent years. Boys desire to clean, but they require guidance in doing so. Ensure you teach teen boys how to shave or trim their hair and other related topics properly.

Hygiene is essential to our daily routine because it ensures that we are healthy and free of various infections and diseases. Be aware of hygiene tips for your teenage boys and apply them. Remember that hygiene never causes harm to anyone.

For Girls

As your daughter grows and changes, hygiene becomes more important. Here's what she should know about personal hygiene, menstruation, and other puberty-related changes.

Personal Care

Knowing the fundamentals of personal hygiene is the first step that every adolescent must take. Assist your adolescent in developing a routine and demonstrating proper skin care. Make it fun with girly body wash, shampoo, and colorful soaps.

Understand the Signs of Puberty

Knowing when your child is approaching puberty can assist you in preparing her for the changes. There will be many changes as your child enters the wonderful world of adolescence. If your daughter reaches puberty before age eight, she may be experiencing precocious puberty. Here's what you should know to assist her in adjusting.

Shaving and Girls

Personal hygiene for girls includes knowing when and how to shave. It takes time to learn how to shave safely, so demonstrate to your daughter how to hold a razor, clean the blade, and prepare the skin with foam or shaving gel.

Pads or Tampons?

Every girl should be able to tell the difference between tampons and pads. Your daughter's hygiene depends on her understanding of how to use the products safely.

Acne

There are challenges even when you practice good personal hygiene. Acne is a natural part of growing up, but that doesn't mean your child has no say. You can assist your adolescent by understanding how acne develops and how to treat it.

Segue: The next chapter will talk about the importance of setting boundaries and discipline.

Chapter 7: I: Instilling Boundaries and Good Behavior

What comes to mind when you think of a boundary? Consider something like a property line or a shape's defining lines. Boundaries indicate where one thing ends and another starts. Boundaries in a relationship work similarly; they help each person determine where one person ends and the other begins. In short, boundaries help you define your comfort zone and how you want to be treated by others. They apply to any relationship, whether it is with a friend, family member, partner, or anyone else in your life.

Setting Healthy Boundaries with Your Teenager

Teens are frequently placed in challenging situations with friends or dating partners where they can't communicate their needs or values. Even if their gut instinct tells them someone is crossing a line with them, they may struggle to express their discomfort. As a result, parents must work with their teenagers to establish boundaries with others. Although boundaries are unique to each individual, when used correctly, they help teens set limits for their protection. Boundaries ease communication with others about what is and is not acceptable to them, which is critical for teen friendships and dating relationships. Boundaries may even be required with specific adult figures in their lives, such as a coach or a relative. Here are some guidelines for assisting your teen in setting boundaries.

What Exactly Are Boundaries?

Teens set boundaries for their protection from hurt, manipulation, or being taken advantage of in some way. Boundaries express self-worth for a teen by letting others know their values and how they prefer to be treated. Furthermore, boundaries create necessary space between a teen and others. Healthy boundaries are essential for the success of any relationship, platonic or romantic. Boundaries help teens understand their feelings and limits and require them to communicate those feelings and limits clearly and honestly.

Why Are Boundaries Important for Teens?

Setting physical and emotional boundaries is an essential part of growing up. It's also necessary for developing respectful, supportive, and healthy friendships and dating relationships. Unfortunately, many teenagers struggle to set boundaries with their friends and in their dating relationships. It puts them at risk for unhealthy friendships, bullying, and dating abuse. Setting boundaries is, of course, a difficult task. It's unsettling and forces teens to assert themselves and draw boundaries. Furthermore, communicating boundaries to others can lead to awkward conversations or situations.

Nonetheless, it is one of the most important things for teenagers to learn. Setting boundaries with others will not only keep your teen safe but also protect their mental health. An unhealthy relationship or dating abuse can have several negative consequences. Your teen should set boundaries with people who make them feel uncomfortable, worthless, or disrespected, such as a controlling partner, fake friends, or an adult. Allowing people to treat them in unhealthy ways leads to unhealthy relationships and can also have a mental and emotional impact on your teen.

How to Establish Boundaries

Teens, like adults, face a variety of different scenarios in their relationships. They may need to inform one friend that they do not want to share their homework and another that they do not want to gossip about other people. Perhaps another friend is particularly bossy, and another constantly borrows money. These are all situations in which setting boundaries can be beneficial. Teens may even find themselves in situations where they must express their feelings about sex or alcohol. The point is that your teen will encounter various situations throughout their life that will test their values and beliefs, and knowing how to set boundaries can help them stay safe while remaining true to themselves.

What to Do When They Break Their Boundaries

Teens break boundaries because they dislike, disagree with, or do not understand them. Pushback from teenagers is expected, and as frustrating as it is for parents, we know that testing the boundaries is a normal part of maturing from adolescence to adulthood.

Understanding Their Reasons

When we face opposition from our children, it's easy to give in to the temptation to back down or relax our boundaries. This is a significant mistake in terms of child development. The more you relax your boundaries when your children push back, the more likely they will try to railroad you. Being "nice" will not get you far. On the other hand, being fair and consistent is the most effective way to nudge your children toward more mature, responsible behavior. Young people require firm boundaries, and when they challenge us and violate the ones we've established, we must continue to enforce them.

For example, if your child disables or deletes the parental controls you've installed on their device, the worst thing you can do is suspend your rules. Parents who dismiss online safety as "too difficult" because "they'll always find a way to get around the system" miss the point. The issue is not with the strategy or tool. It's about the breaking of rules. We would never consider removing speed limits simply because people only sometimes obey them. Instead, we establish clear penalties for breaking the rules.

Discipline Strategies

Discipline does not imply punishment. It is about guiding children in appropriate behavior. Discipline for pre-teens and teenagers entails agreeing on and setting appropriate limits and assisting them in adhering to those limits. You most likely used a variety of discipline strategies when your child was younger to teach them the fundamentals of good behavior. As your child enters adolescence, you can use limits and boundaries to help them learn independence, accept responsibility for their actions and the consequences, and solve problems. These skills are required for your child to develop into a young adult with standards for appropriate behavior and respect for others. An essential part is learning to follow explicit rules agreed upon in advance.

Use Consequences as a Form of Adolescent Discipline

Your child may occasionally test your limits or violate the rules you've established. Consequences are one way to deal with this. This is how.

Make the Outcome Appropriate

If you tailor the punishment to the misbehavior, your child will be more likely to consider the issue. It may also feel more equitable to your child. For example, if your child arrives home later than agreed, a practical consequence could be having to arrive home earlier the next time.

Withdraw Your Cooperation

This strategy is intended to help your child understand your point of view and learn that they must give and take. It also teaches your child that every action has a consequence. Your child can reap the benefits of doing the right thing. However, doing the wrong thing results in a negative outcome. Inform your child that you may withdraw your cooperation due to misbehavior. 'If you want me to iron your shirt for tonight, you must speak respectfully to me,' for example. Saying you're willing to follow through on a consequence can sometimes be enough to influence behavior.

Withdraw Permissions

This consequence should be used with caution. It will only work well if you use it sparingly. The idea is to take away something you know your child enjoys, such as visits to a friend's house, technology access, or activities. You must inform your child ahead of time that this is your intention so that they can decide whether losing the privilege is worthwhile. This consequence does not require you to withdraw privileges for an extended period. Aim for a temporary withdrawal within a few days of the misbehavior.

What Does Respect Mean to a Teenager?

Your relationships are held together by respect. Learn how to be respectful and what to do when someone disrespects you. Respect for others is essential because it allows us to feel safe and express ourselves. Growing up and having important people respect us teaches us how to respect others. Respecting someone means accepting them wholly, regardless of your differences. Respect builds trust, safety, and well-being in relationships. Respect does not have to come naturally; it can be learned. Respect for others is one piece of the puzzle. It is also essential to respect yourself. Remember that you are valuable and vital. What you think and feel is as important as what others think and feel. Ending an unrespectful relationship is a way of respecting yourself.

How to Teach Them to Respect

Demanding respect is ineffective. It is ineffective to remind teenagers that you have already taught them respect. Do you want to learn how to teach your adolescent respect? It is by respecting your adolescent. What they receive, they will return. But how do you show them respect when they don't deserve it? Try these simple but effective ways to get started, and your teenager won't mind!

Before Entering, Knock on the Door

I know it's not a revolutionary concept, and it's "your house," but teenagers crave their personal space. Knocking and waiting for their response shows respect for his privacy. You can patiently wait for the green light to enter while he is dressing or is not ready to see people for whatever reason. Knocking indicates that you recognize his maturation and, as a result, respect his privacy.

Ask For Her Opinion and Then Follow It

Not every time, but at least once in a while, solicit your teen's opinion and then act on it. Teenagers believe that adults never value their opinions or dismiss them as inferior. Despite having more life experience than our teens, they can still have a great idea or a valid opinion worth acting on now and then. So, whenever possible, take advantage of it. They will be astounded—and validated. Considering her opinion shows her that you value her thoughts and ideas.

Give Her More Time to Complete Her Chores

When I ask my children to do something, I expect them to do it immediately. There is also value in teaching children to obey right away. On the other hand, teens have more responsibilities and frequently have agendas. Consider giving her a larger time frame to complete the task. Instead of taking out the garbage right now, ask her to take it out before dinner tonight. If she appears to be busy, ask, "When would you like to take care of this?" Being more flexible does not imply that you are making the task optional; instead, it demonstrates to your teen that you value her time.

Allow Him to Choose His Bedtime and Wake-Up Time

It is difficult for those who like to have control to delegate bedtime and wake-up time to our teenagers. We must deal with the consequences when they stay up too late and are tired the next day. On the other hand, a teen can learn a lot by managing their sleep schedule. He'll learn that getting through the school day and sports practice is challenging if you've only slept for four hours five days in a row. And when he puts off homework until the last minute, the price is either a long, arduous night or a low grade. These things are usually pretty good teachers, albeit challenging to observe. Allowing him to manage his bedtime demonstrates that you value his ability to learn from his choices.

Allow Him a Privilege That His Younger Siblings Do Not Have

We frequently expect a lot from older children since they are more capable. The youngest child must clear their plate after eating, and the oldest child does the dishes. The oldest children must also deal with more homework, complex relationships, and possibly their first paid jobs. Being the oldest may appear to be a disadvantage—unless you give him privileges the younger children don't have, such as staying out later. Treating a teen as an adult demonstrates that you value his age and family position.

I understand how difficult it is to show your teenagers respect when you don't believe they deserve it. So approach it as an experiment. Choose just one of these and observe how it affects your relationship. Instead of lecturing or demanding respect, demonstrate it to your child. They will want to respect you.

How Boys Must Respect Women

Boys must learn the value of respect to grow into well-rounded men. Teaching your son to respect women begins at a young age, and your influence as a parent is critical. The example will influence your son's perception of the respect you set at home, such as the bond between a mother and son or the respect a father shows his wife. Here are some suggestions for teaching your son to respect women.

Teach Your Son How to Form Healthy Relationships With Women

The importance of encouraging young boys to form positive friendships with girls cannot be over-emphasized. The sooner this is accomplished, the more at ease they will be around girls, allowing them to see past teenage boys' stereotypes about girls. Early friendships between boys and girls encourages lifelong mutual respect.

Emphasize the Significance of Consent

Boys must respect her when she says "no" and should not touch her without her permission. Teach your son that consent conversations should be repeated during intimacy and practice scenarios in which this would occur.

Women Should Be Treated With Respect

Remember to consider the influence of your example. Your son needs to see respect in his family, friendships, and all situations. Listen to and respect women's opinions as parents. When addressing women, use respectful terms, manners, and body language, and surround your son with positive role models.

Keep Track of His Media Consumption

Allowing your son to watch content that is not age-appropriate or glorifies violence should be avoided. According to psychologist Dr. Justin Coulson, this type of content desensitizes children and reduces their penchant for showing empathy and kindness. Remind your son that depicting women as one-dimensional objects in movies, games, and other forms of media is not accurate or reflective of reality. Discuss with your son how pornography devalues women and why he should avoid it. Set appropriate internet parental controls and empower him to say no when exposed to this content.

How Parents Can Respect Their Teens

Teens frequently make the error of equating respect with permission. "If you respect me, you'll let me," they say. Is that what your son is telling you? If so, you should be aware that this is not the case. Respect and permission are not the same things. You are the parent, and your child must respect your authority and follow your rules as long as he lives with you.

What is the definition of "respect"? And how does it work in the context of a relationship between two people who are not "equal" in terms of position and authority? Respect between parent and child is best defined as giving a person the special attention or regard he deserves. It's a matter of demonstrating that you hold him in high regard. It is always critical to give your son "special attention" and "special regard," even though he is a minor. However, if you follow these helpful hints, you will be able to complete the task successfully.

Before drawing conclusions or making decisions, give your teen your full attention. Take as much time as you need. It might or might not change your mind, but first, listen. Listening does not imply agreement. Trust him as far as he has proven himself trustworthy. Trust must be earned. Allow your son as much freedom as he has demonstrated he can handle. Nothing more, nothing less. This can be a tricky balancing act.

Maintain consistency in your words, actions, decisions, rules, and choices. A teenager finds it difficult to respect someone who is inconsistent or hypocritical. Make rules that are logical, fair, reasonable, and true. Rules are frequently created for the parent's convenience, to assuage an adult's fears, or to satisfy his need for control. Refuse the temptation. Recognize when he is correct and you are incorrect. Mutual respect is built on such openness. Never make fun of or intentionally embarrass him. It makes no difference whether you do it publicly or privately. Even if you're angry, don't call people names.

Parents' careless words can cause serious harm to children. Differentiate between behavior and character. It's one thing to point out wrongdoing, but avoid attacking your child's character. Remind him that he is made in the image of God. This is fundamental to what it means to be human. And if your son is a Christian—if he claims to be a representative of the Lord—he should seek the respect of others as a way of honoring God through his witness.

You'll be showing him respect if you do these things regularly, even if you can't always "give in" to his requests. This balance of justice, guidance, and respect will serve as a useful example of how he should respect you even when you disagree.

How to Talk to Them About Body Image

Body image refers to how a person sees themselves in the mirror and how they feel in and about their body, and it does not always accurately reflect the perspectives of others. Teens can feel extremely vulnerable, uncomfortable, or self-conscious about their bodies due to physical changes during puberty and uneven physical development happening during this time, whether considered overweight medically or by society.

Teens struggle during adolescence because they don't understand how physiological changes in their bodies affect weight and fat distribution. Parents must encourage their teenagers to be as at ease in their skin as possible. Parents can have a strong influence—both positive and negative—on their teens' positive body image formation and maintenance. Ways that parents can influence their children's perceptions of themselves include the following:

Don't Allow Yourself to Be Seduced by Cultural and Media Body Image Standards

Make it a point to mention that different people, eras, and cultures have different beauty standards. Hollywood has yet to have a single confirmed and definitive definition of what constitutes attractiveness.

Consider Your Options Before Speaking

Directly confronting a teen about their body and weight can be problematic if done without tact. For example, a well-intentioned parent who tells her child regularly that she is concerned about the child's weight can hurt the teen's body image. Over time, this can encourage a disordered eating pattern to meet the parent's bodily standards.

Reduce Triggers

The discomfort regarding a negative body image may happen when the teen is weighed at the doctor's office or while shopping for clothes. Parents can avoid focusing on appearance or weight by emphasizing other aspects where their teen shines, such as talents, positive characteristics, or passions.

Address Weight Gain or Loss With Caution

Many parents struggle with how to talk to their teenagers about weight gain or loss in a sensitive manner. If you notice your teen is gaining weight or has gone up several clothing sizes (or is losing weight and needs a smaller size), try to maintain a neutral tone and ask how your teen feels about changes in their body. Continue the conversation based on your teen's response. Similarly, if you or your teen's physician had recommended weight loss to your teen and they see "positive" results, maintain a neutral tone and ask your teen how they feel.

Finally, remind your teen that their health and happiness should not be equated with weight loss, gain, or overall appearance. Instead, your teen must strike a balance between focusing on their talents, passions, strengths, and other valuable qualities and focusing on appearance.

Eating Disorders

For teenagers, having an eating disorder such as anorexia is a severe problem. Refusing to eat or severely restricting food intake harms their health and can be fatal if not treated. Even with that looming threat, an adolescent with anorexia will struggle to gain the weight required to survive. Instead, they will do whatever it takes to avoid gaining weight, such as excessive calorie counting, extreme exercising, avoiding dinner time, throwing away food, etc.

These are the symptoms of their disease, which are upsetting for parents to witness. Parents of anorexic teenagers are frequently surprised when their otherwise healthy child enters early adolescence and becomes food-avoidant to the point of starvation. Anorectic adolescent parents may feel baffled and helpless; they may also blame themselves, believing they must have done something to cause their child's problems.

What Aids Parents in Supporting Their Anorexic Children

Parents may not need special skills to assist their children. However, they need to understand a few things about their child's condition and gain confidence in themselves when it comes to getting their child to eat. First, parents must recognize that they did not cause their child's disease and will not be held accountable for it. This message needs to be reinforced because there are so many societal messages out there that say parents are to blame for their child's mental health problems that it can be difficult for parents to let go of that notion.

Second, parents must understand that anorexia is a disease and not blame it on their child. Anorexic children aren't rebellious or punishing their parents. They are just entrapped by anxieties, fears, and behaviors, and they require assistance breaking free.

Third, parents require assurance that they can learn with the help of a therapist how to assist their child in changing their eating habits. Many parents bring their children to therapy after several failed attempts to get them to eat, leaving them feeling helpless and anxious. One goal of treatment is to help parents see that they already have the skills necessary to do what needs to be done. Getting a child to eat is like that of a nurse administering medication to a patient—someone who does not accept "no" for an answer and does not negotiate.

Teenagers and Depression

Every adolescent experiences sadness or mood swings. When a teen's sad or lousy mood lasts for weeks or longer, and there are other changes in how they act, this could be a sign of depression. With the right therapy, depression is treatable. However, if problems are not addressed, they can persist or worsen. Teens who are depressed require additional support from their parents and other adults in their lives and therapy. Talk to your teen if you suspect they are depressed. Tell them you want to know what they're going through. If they want to talk, they should listen.

Is My Adolescent Depressed?

While mood swings and acting out are common during adolescence, depression is a different story. It has far-reaching consequences that go beyond a depressed mood. Depression destroys a teen's essence, leading to overwhelming sadness, despair, or anger. Most rebellious and unhealthy behaviors or attitudes in teens may be signs of depression. The following are some examples of how teenagers "act out" in an attempt to cope with emotional pain:

- persistent bad mood

- issues at school

- disinterest in activities

- getting away

- abuse of drugs and alcohol

- addiction to smartphones

What Should I Do if I Believe My Adolescent Is Depressed?

If you suspect your adolescent is depressed, take the following steps:

Speak With Them

Extend your love and support. Let them know you care and want to hear about their problems. Many depressed teenagers feel isolated, distant, or unlovable. Small acts of kindness can make them feel less alone.

Take Them to the Doctor

Make an appointment for your teen to see their doctor or a mental health provider to screen for depression. Medical professionals can also investigate other health or mental health issues that may be causing your teen's symptoms. They can tell you how they and you can help your teen.

Anxiety in Teens

We, as parents, always want the best for our children. When faced with life's challenges, we want them to be healthy, happy, and resilient. Anxiety is common in teenagers and manifests itself at various stages of development. Anxiety disorders are diagnosed in children as young as four years old, and approximately 32% of adolescents in the United States have an anxiety disorder (Newport Academy,

2020b). This figure has steadily increased over the years. According to the study, one in every four to five adolescents has a severe disability due to their anxiety disorder.

Parents face a challenging moment handling a teen with anxiety. The good news is that the condition is highly treatable. There is also a lot you can do to assist your child. Don't assume that your child will naturally overcome their anxiety. Begin taking steps to help your teen manage the symptoms and to regain control over how they perceive the world around them.

Anxiety Symptoms in Teenagers

Anxiety symptoms vary greatly and are frequently misdiagnosed in children and adolescents. The majority of teenagers' concerns are related to their feelings about themselves. These may include academic performance and pressures to succeed in school, how others perceive them, and body image concerns related to physical development. Teens' anxiety is not always apparent because they conceal their thoughts and feelings. Some warning signs to look for include the following:

- constant worries or fears about mundane aspects of their lives

- withdrawal from social activities or friends

- irritation or lashing out at others

- difficulties at school or a drop in performance

- refusal to attend school

- sleep issues

- abuse of substances

- always looking for reassurance

How to Talk to a Teen About Anxiety

Assure your teen that, in certain situations, anxiety can be a protective emotion. Anxiety alerts us to potential dangers and keeps us safe. That uneasy feeling in the gut that we all get from time to time could be a warning sign of a potential threat. Because paying attention to these warning signs can help you avoid dangerous situations, feeling anxious can be beneficial. You can also help your teen feel less anxious by discussing what they can do to improve a specific situation in the future.

Maintain an open line of communication with your teen. Maintaining effective communication with teenagers can be difficult, if not unpleasant, at times. Teenagers will only sometimes confide in their parents as they become more independent. A supportive communication style will increase trust and comfort when sharing emotions. Maintaining regular contact with teenagers and inquiring about their day is critical. They may not go into great detail, but they will recognize your genuine interest and concern for them. A few words of encouragement can go a long way. Tell your teen you're proud of them and their progress. If they express concern or anxiety about a specific situation, this is an opportunity to start a more in-depth discussion. Phrases such as "I know this is a difficult situation" or "that sounds very hurtful" validate their feelings.

Make use of active listening skills. Teens look to their parents for supportive connections and outlets for their emotions. You can help them feel less anxious by listening carefully and validating their feelings without passing judgment or criticism. Giving your teen your full attention and making eye contact shows interest in what they're saying, and occasionally nodding shows that you're truly listening. Avoid interrupting your teen while speaking so they can express themselves completely.

Teens and Bullying

Bullying is typically characterized by intent, repetition, and power. A bully repeatedly wants to cause pain through physical harm, hurtful words, or behavior. Boys are usually physically bullied, while girls face psychological bullying. It's a behavioral pattern, not a single incident. Bullies usually have an assumed high social status or position of power, such as being bigger, stronger, or popular.

Bullying is more likely to affect the most vulnerable children. It can occur in person or online. Bullying on social media, SMS/text or instant message, email, or any other online platform where children interact is standard. Because parents may not continuously monitor what their children do on these platforms, it can be challenging to determine when their child has been impacted.

Why Should I Step In if My Child Is Being Bullied?

Bullying can have long-term adverse effects on children. Aside from physical consequences, children who are bullied suffer emotionally and mentally, such as depression and anxiety. These lead to substance abuse and poor academic performance. Unlike in-person bullying, online bullying reaches a victim anytime and anywhere. It can potentially cause significant harm because it quickly reaches a large audience and leaves a permanent online footprint for everyone involved. Your child has the right to attend school in a safe, nurturing environment that respects their dignity.

What Should I Do if My Child Is Being Bullied?

If you suspect your child is being bullied, you can take the following steps to assist them:

Openly and calmly listen to your child. Instead of attempting to identify the source of the bullying or to solve the problem, concentrate on making them feel heard and supported. Assure them that it is not their fault. Tell the child that you believe them, that you're glad they told you, that it's not their fault, and that you'll do everything you can to find help.

Speak with the teacher or the school. You and your child are not alone in dealing with bullying. Inquire about your school's bullying policy or code of conduct. This may apply to both in-person and online bullying. Be a pillar of strength. Having a supportive parent is critical for your child in dealing with the effects of bullying. Assure them they can talk to you anytime and that things will improve.

What if My Child Is Bullying Other Children?

If you suspect or know your child is bullying other children, remember that they are not inherently evil and may act out for various reasons. Bullying children frequently want to fit in, need attention, or are simply figuring out how to deal with difficult emotions. Bullies are sometimes victims or witnesses to violence at home or in their community. You should take the following steps to help your child stop bullying:

Communicate

Understanding why your child is acting out will assist you in determining how to assist them. Do they have a sense of insecurity at school? Is it a fight with a friend or a sibling? If they have difficulty explaining their behavior, you may consult a child-oriented counselor, social worker, or mental health professional.

Examine Healthy Coping Strategies

Ask your child to describe a situation that irritated them and offer constructive solutions. Encourage your child to empathize with the one they are bullying. Remind your child that online comments can still cause harm in the real world.

Provide Consequences and Opportunities for Restitution

If you discover that your child has been bullying others, it is critical that you impose appropriate, nonviolent consequences. This limits activities that promote bullying during social gatherings or on social media. Encourage your child to apologize to their peers and think about ways to be more inclusive.

Alcohol and Substance Abuse

It is critical to talk to teenagers about drugs and alcohol. Teens require structure to stay safe. Having clear drug and alcohol policies can be beneficial. You cannot ensure that your rules will not be broken. However, studies show that children with clear rules, even if broken, are less likely to get into serious trouble than children without.

But it cannot be easy to know what to say. Refrain from surprising the kids with a big speech. Instead, tell your child you want to discuss drugs and alcohol with them. Make your rules clear and specific about what will happen if your children break them. Children perform best when they know what to expect. And, if your child is pushed to do something they don't want to, clear rules make it easier for them to say no. Respect conveys that you trust them to act responsibly for your benefit and theirs.

Help your child understand why drinking or using drugs is dangerous and how poor decisions can affect their life. Be truthful and reasonable. Allow children to express their concerns and feelings. They might have hoped for an opportunity to ask questions or check in on something concerning. Inform them that your goal is to keep them safe. Make sure your child understands that they can call you for help in any situation.

Segue: The next chapter will talk about nurturing healthy relationships.

Chapter 8: N: Nurturing Relationships

Open, non-judgmental family discussions without mockery and snide remarks from siblings are needed to encourage a teenager to open up to you. Do you provide such an environment of honesty and complete transparency?

Relationships and Romance for Teenagers

Romantic relationships are a significant developmental stage. These relationships occur alongside adolescence's physical, social, and emotional changes. They are linked to pre-teens' and teenagers' explorations of body image, independence, privacy, and identity. For some young people, these relationships may also include exploring their sexual orientation. Romantic relationships can cause many emotional ups and downs for your child and, in some cases, the entire family. However, these emotions guide your child toward a greater capacity to care, share, and form intimate relationships.

When Pre-teen and Adolescent Romance and Relationships Begin

There is no such thing as a "right" age to begin dating. However, changes frequently occur around these ages:

- Your child may begin to show more independence from her family and interest in friends between the ages of 9 and 11.

- Your child may feel attracted to others between 10 and 14.

- Romantic relationships can become central to adolescent social lives between the ages of 15 and 19.

It's also common for kids to be uninterested in romantic relationships until they're in their late teens. Some young people concentrate on schoolwork, sports, or other activities.

First Loves

Before your child begins dating, they may have one or more crushes. When your child discovers someone they admire and aspire to be like, they have an identity crush. The beginning of romantic feelings is a romantic crush. It's about your child seeing someone else as perfect or ideal. This can reveal what your child finds appealing in other people. Romantic crushes rarely last long because ideals often crumble as your child gets to know the other person better. However, your child's intense feelings are genuine, so take crushes seriously and do not make fun of them.

Relationships in the Pre-Teen and Adolescent Years

Younger teenagers typically hang out in groups. They may meet up with someone special among friends and then gradually spend more time alone with that person. Relationships may last only a few weeks or months during these years. If your child wishes to go out alone with someone special, discussing it with them can help you determine whether they are ready. Is your child looking for a partner because their friends are? Is your child convinced that this is the only way to have fun? Is your child interested in getting to know someone better?

If your child is interested in someone older or younger, it is worth noting that people of different ages may have different expectations from relationships. The adults in their lives are influential role models in the lives of teenagers. Treating your partner, friends, and family with care and respect makes you a positive role model who inspires respectful relationships. Speaking respectfully about people of all genders and sexual orientations teaches your child that everyone is equal and valuable.

Adolescent Same-Sex Attraction and Relationships

Some teens' adolescent sexual development includes same-sex attraction and relationships. While some teenagers develop a bisexual attraction, others are clear about their feelings and who they are attracted to. Some are perplexed when their feelings and attractions differ from those of their friends or what they see in the media. Responding positively and nonjudgmentally is an excellent first step in either case. If you are having difficulty remaining calm and positive, find another adult whom you and your child trust and with whom your child can pray and discuss their feelings.

Sex and Adolescent Relationships

If your child is in a relationship, it may raise issues of sex and intimacy. Not all adolescent relationships involve sex, but most will experiment with sexual behavior at some point. As a result, your child requires specific information about consent, contraception, safe sex, and STDs. This could also be an opportunity to discuss dealing with unwanted sexual and peer pressure. If you let your child know you're available to listen, they will likely come to you with questions or concerns.

Discussing Romance, Relationships, and Sex with Teenagers

When you encourage conversations in your family about feelings, friendships, and family relationships, your child will feel more confident discussing adolescent relationships. If your child understands what respectful relationships entail, they can apply this directly to romantic relationships. These conversations may indicate that your child will feel more comfortable sharing their feelings with you as they develop romantic feelings for others. These conversations can also bring up other important topics, such as treating others with kindness, breaking up with kindness, and respecting others' boundaries.

Talking about sex and relationships with your child from a young age may make them more comfortable asking you questions as they enter adolescence. Discussing romantic and sexual adolescent relationships is similar to discussing friendships or attending a party. You and your child may need to discuss behavior, ground rules, and consequences for breaking the rules, depending on your values and family rules. You could, for example, discuss how much time your child spends with their partner versus how much time they spend studying or whether it is acceptable for their partner to stay over.

Dealing with Breakups in Adolescent Relationships

Breakups and broken hearts are common in adolescent relationships. Worse, teenage breakups, such as at school or on social media, may occur publicly. You can expect your child to become depressed and emotional when their relationship ends. This may not appear to be the case, but it is part of learning how to deal with difficult decisions and disappointments. Your child may require time and space, a shoulder to cry on, and an open ear to listen. Your child may also require some distraction.

Relationships for Disabled Pre-Teens and Teenagers

Pre-teens and teenagers with disabilities have the same interest and need for information about romance, relationships, and intimacy as other teenagers. Sexual activity rates for young people with disabilities are comparable to those of other teenagers. Ensure that your child receives developmentally appropriate sex education at home and school. Your health professional, local community resources, and relevant support groups should all be able to assist you.

Are They in a Healthy Relationship?

In the early stages of a relationship, it's perfectly normal to see the world through rose-colored glasses. However, for some people, rose-colored glasses become blinders, preventing them from seeing that a relationship isn't as healthy as it should be. Hopefully, your teen and their significant other are taking good care of each other. They should take a step back from the dizzying sensation of being swept off their feet and consider whether their relationship possesses the following characteristics:

Mutual Admiration

Is he or she aware of how amazing you are and why? Make sure your boyfriend or girlfriend likes you for who you are. Does your partner listen when you say you're unsure about something and then back off? Respect in a relationship implies that each person values the other and understands—and would never test—the other's boundaries.

Trust

While you talk with a guy from French class, your boyfriend walks by. Is he going to lose his cool because he lacks trust? It's normal to feel jealous occasionally; jealousy is a natural emotion. What matters is how a person reacts when they are jealous. You can't have a healthy relationship if you don't trust each other.

Excellent Communication.

Can you communicate with each other and share your feelings? Don't keep your emotions bottled up because you're afraid they'll offend your boyfriend or girlfriend. And if you need time to think about something before you're ready to talk about it, the right person will give you that time.

Honesty

This one is related to trust because it's difficult to trust someone when one of you isn't being honest. Have you ever caught your girlfriend in the act of telling a big lie? Like she told you she had to work on Friday night but ended up going to the movies with her friends? You'll have much more difficulty believing her the next time she says she has to work, and your trust will be on shaky ground.

Keep Your Identities Separate

Everyone in a healthy relationship must make sacrifices. But that doesn't mean you should feel like you are losing your identity. You both had your own lives when you started going out (families, friends, interests, hobbies, etc.), which should not change. Neither of you should be forced to pretend to like something you don't, to forego seeing your friends, or to abandon activities you enjoy. You should also feel free to continue developing new skills or interests, making new friends, and progressing.

Fairness/Equality

You need to have give-and-take in your relationship. Do you take turns choosing which new movie to see? As a couple, do you hang out with your partner's friends as often as you do with yours? You'll know if it isn't a pretty fair balance. Things get bad fast when a relationship turns into a power struggle, with one person fighting to get their way all the time.

Why Is Teenage Love So Intense?

Teens' relationships can be more intense because they are hypersensitive to what others think of them and lack a broader perspective gained through experience. Teens, for example, are more likely than adults to assume personal rejection rather than "life happens" as an explanation if a love interest does not call when they say they will. Another source of intensity is adolescents' "all-in" impulsivity: teens may lack inhibitory abilities because their executive brain functioning is still developing. Given their own romantic love experiences, parents may dismiss their teen's feelings or compare teen and adult romantic love. Instead, they can use the experience to teach others.

How Are Teenagers Affected by Relationships?

Changes in a teen's physical and mental development are accompanied by significant changes in their relationships with family and friends. During puberty, family relationships are frequently reorganized. Teens want more independence and emotional distance from their parents. A teen's attention is frequently drawn to social interactions and friendships. This includes friends of the same gender, friends of the same gender in groups, and friends of different genders. Interest in dating and sexual relationships is triggered by sexual maturity.

Peer Relationships

Teens spend more time with their peers. They report that their friends have made them feel more understood and accepted. Parents and other family members are receiving less and less attention. Teens with similar interests, social classes, and ethnic backgrounds tend to form close friendships. While childhood friendships are often based on shared interests, teen friendships can include shared attitudes, values, and activities. Educational interests are also common in teen friendships.

Close and intimate self-disclosing discussions with friends, particularly with girls, allow for exploring identities and defining a teen's sense of self. Conversations within these meaningful friendships also assist teenagers in exploring their sexuality and their feelings about it. Teenage boys' friendships are frequently less intimate than those of teenage girls. Boys' friends usually validate each other's worth through actions and deeds rather than personal sharing.

Male-Female Relationships

Sexual interest and social and cultural influences and expectations influence the shift to male-female and sexual relationships. Observation and practice are used to learn social and cultural expectations and behaviors in male-female or sexual relationships. Developmental tasks during adolescence include struggles to control sexual and aggressive urges. It is also possible to discover potential or actual love relationships.

During adolescence, sexual behaviors include impulsive behavior, various experimental interactions for mutual exploring, and intercourse. Males and females have different expectations of sexual and love relationships due to biological differences and differences in how they socialize. These factors influence sexual escapades and influence teens' future sexual actions and partnerships. Over time, a mutually fulfilling sexual partnership in a love relationship may be discovered.

How to Talk to Them About Heartache

Teens' emotions are solid and strange, and they must deal with new interoceptive signaling as their physiology changes. Contrary to popular belief, boys are more likely than girls to experience mental distress due to heartbreak. Teens benefit from their parents' understanding and support in coping with this trauma. When a teen's first love ends, parents interpret the loss through the myths that their grief is fleeting and that, during the acute phase, girls are more vulnerable to the impact of love grief than boys.

Differences Between Boys and Girls During a Breakup

Girls are said to be more reliant on close relationships than boys, so a breakup is expected to hurt them more. However, this is just one of many common assumptions about what girls and boys feel that turn out to be false. When it comes to romantic relationships, teenage girls are less vulnerable than teen boys after a breakup. Those working on the front lines of adolescent mental health have known for many years that "The boys fall apart when they break up with a girlfriend," a high school counselor explained. "They are unable to study. They [occasionally] begin to drink. I can assist them if they come to me with problems at work or with their parents. But I see a red flag when they say they've just broken up with a girlfriend."

The difference is that girls have a more extensive social network to draw from. Close friends act as emotional co-regulators; they help them reflect on their feelings through intimate conversations, stimulating the brain's executive functions and calming anxiety and despair. Boys rely more on a romantic partner, who may be their sole source of intimacy. They tend to end friendship intimacy in later adolescence as the guy code desires strength, independence, and carrying emotional burdens silently. Furthermore, boys have more stable friendships and are less experienced in the brutal lessons of rupture and repair that girls learn in late childhood. A first romantic breakup becomes a trauma that takes a long time to process.

This distinction can be seen in the language used by teenagers to describe their experiences. Teenage girls describe breakups as "really hard" or "a shock" and admit to feeling "lost" or "stuck." In contrast, teenage boys use words like "falling apart," "shipwrecked," and "tailspin," which imply severe disruption and disorientation. The rejection of a lover jeopardizes their identity, health, and mood. Nobody should add to their loneliness by downplaying their suffering.

How To Help Your Teen Deal with a Breakup

The end of a relationship, whether it's a first true love or a summer fling, is emotionally draining for a teen who is still learning about heartbreak. They're flying high on the wings of love one minute, then crash into a sea of heartache the next. Fortunately, a breakup can teach your teen how to manage pain, rejection, or disappointment when a relationship ends. Of course, you also want to avoid situations that could aggravate your teen's distress.

Validate Your Teen's Feelings

Resist the urge to downplay your child's feelings; just because you didn't think the relationship was that important or would last forever doesn't mean your adolescent didn't care about their ex. While it's unlikely they would have lived happily ever after, your teen may have believed they would. Regardless, your teen's pain is real and significant. Validate your teen's feelings by saying things like, "I know this is difficult," or "I know it's sad when a relationship ends." Avoid phrases such as "this isn't a big deal" or "high school relationships don't usually work out anyway." Comments to soothe the pain may end up making your teen feel isolated or misunderstood. You may believe your teen's heartache is determined by gender, but avoid these assumptions.

Support Their Decision

Even if your teen initiated the breakup, that doesn't mean they won't be upset. Sometimes the person who chooses to end the relationship is the most heartbroken. However, if the breakup occurs, support your child. If you like their significant other, don't try to talk them out of the breakup. And don't say they made the wrong decision. This is your teen's relationship, so even if you think it's a bad idea to end it, let your teen make that decision. You can help them work through their feelings and understand why they ended the relationship.

Find a Middle Ground

Your first instinct may be to shower your child with well-intended, reassuring statements like "you can do better" or "they weren't right for you anyway." You'll probably want to tell them they're too young to be so serious, or you'll resort to the ultimate relationship cliché: "There are plenty of fish in the sea." However, these sentiments are generally ineffective. Saying "I told you so" about a partner you warned them about is neither helpful nor supportive. Criticizing your teen's ex will almost certainly make them feel even worse. And they're more likely to be defensive and less willing to confide in you.

Be an Effective Listener

Allowing your teen to speak without interjecting your opinions or analysis is better than saying anything. Your teen does not need you to take charge, tell them how they should feel, or tell them what you would do or feel if you were in their shoes. They need time and a safe space to express their frustration, confusion, and hurt without anyone second-guessing or clouding their judgment. They don't need you to filter their emotions or put them in context; time will do that for them.

Discuss Technology

Nowadays, some teenagers rush to update their relationship status and share details about their lives on social media. Talk to your teen about taking a technology break in the days or perhaps weeks after breaking up so they don't post updates they'll regret—or end up getting online shaming or backlash. Warn them, in particular, against bad-mouthing ex-partners, posting personal details of the breakup, or sharing anything personal learned during the relationship.

Teens frequently lack the maturity to understand how to handle a breakup respectfully. They may require your assistance in making sound decisions regarding public disclosure of the relationship (and its demise).

Provide Some Distraction

Nothing like creating a distraction to take your child's mind off their breakup. Take them out for a day of fun. You could go to a movie, shopping, or a baseball game. Take them out to their favorite restaurant or make a special dessert together. Consider your teen's favorite activities and plan them out for the day. Or they can collaborate on a project such as planting a garden, creating a scrapbook, experimenting with art supplies, or redecorating their bedroom. Activity keeps your teen away from social media and reminds them that life is pretty good even if they don't have a boyfriend or girlfriend.

Maintain Your Teen's Attention

Remember to keep one thing in mind throughout this process: This is not your breakup. While you may have adored or despised your teen's ex-boyfriend or girlfriend, keep your emotions out of the matter in the best way possible. Teen love is bumpy, and you don't want to be caught off guard if the two reconcile down the road. Furthermore, you don't want your child to feel burdened by having to assist you in dealing with your feelings and their own.

Your priority should be to assist your child in coping with and learning from this experience. They will most likely emerge stronger, more confident, and more mature. For the time being, remind them of how smart, kind, loved, and wonderful they are. Tell them how much you adore them.

Teen love can be exhilarating, but teen heartbreak can be devastating. Support your child during this challenging time by showing them love, patience, and compassion. Recognize that you do not need to save them from their emotions. Feeling these painful emotions is an essential part of the healing process. Being present for your teen is as simple as listening with love and allowing them to heal.

Segue: The next chapter will talk about preparing yourself and your kid for college and leaving home.

CHAPTER 9: G: GET SET GO!

Are you anxious about your kid going out into the world alone? Do you worry about their college and future? These are difficult decisions to make. It's time you remind these almost-adults that you're still available to talk about anything: College...money ...tuition fees...loans...separation anxiety.

How College Changes the Parent/Child Relationship

College is a formative time for students' minds and life skills. College may be the first time for hundreds of thousands of undergrads in the United States who enroll as teenagers to manage their schedules and master a laundry routine. College is also a watershed moment in students' relationships with their parents. Many undergrads, particularly those who live on campus, are caught between dependence and independence, making their own rules and schedules but relying on their parents to help them apply for financial aid and health insurance. They also do their own grocery shopping, but their parents are still likely to foot the bill; they may live in a dorm, but their home is still likely to be their parents' house, to which they return on breaks and during the summer. And this limbo may spur a healthy evolution in students' relationships with their parents.

Parent-child relationships are typically among the most enduring of the close relationships people form in their lifetime. People's "understanding of parents"—their perception of them as real people—was found to be low in their late teens and early twenties and then rose through late adulthood. Adolescents are especially prone to having negative opinions about their parents. This is due in part to adolescents' desire for parental emancipation to establish social autonomy and their identity.

Cradle to College

Despite the myth that American higher education is an all-inclusive time for freedom, exploration, and no responsibility beyond studying, nearly four million college students in the United States are also parents. Roughly one-fifth of all undergraduates do not include students who may be caring for other family members while pursuing a degree. A narrow conception of college, in which everyone earns a four-year degree in four years, persists, as does an even narrower perception of who college students are. According to the Lumina Foundation (Today's Student, n.d.), 37% of college students are 25 or older, 46% are first-generation students, and most work while attending classes.

With so little support for young parents and so few resources to be both a successful parent and a successful student, the current American education system appears to send a message to parenting students that they don't belong on college campuses. That begs the larger question: What kind of young person gets to dream about the future first?

Title IX prohibits schools from discriminating against students based on their "pregnant or parenting status." Nonetheless, young parents are frequently subjected to exclusionary educational policies, such as attendance policies that penalize them for medical absences or being placed in alternative education programs that isolate them from peers.

Some programs assist student parents and some institutions, such as community colleges, provide more flexibility for parents than a four-year school might. In fact, according to Cruse and colleagues (2019), student parents are most likely to attend community college. Community college funding is critical for addressing the complexities of students' lives and preparing them for success. According to a 2021 Generation Hope report based on focus groups, holistic support for student parents at community colleges and four-year schools varies by institution. Community colleges must have the resources to provide support to reimagine what higher education can be and who has access to it. Nonetheless, policymakers need to see or recognize parenting students more.

How to Help Them with Their College Decision

Your role will change as your student assumes adult responsibilities, but your student will still require your assistance. Students rely on you to help them grow, develop, and be independent and a stable force in their ever-changing world. They may need your advice occasionally but not ask for it. Learning to navigate this difficult time can be challenging, rewarding, frightening, and even humorous for you and your student. Advice and additional resources are provided below to assist you throughout your student's educational journey.

Checking-In

Allow your students to share their feelings or ideas as they experience new viewpoints or perspectives challenging the old systems. Let your student explore ideas with an open mind. Acknowledge that differences in viewpoints, dressing, behavior, eating or sleeping habits, and relationships with parents are normal during college.

Telling Your Student That "These Are the Best Years of Your Life" Is Not a Good Idea.

The first year of college can be filled with uncertainty, insecurity, disappointment, and, most importantly, mistakes. It's also full of surprises, inspiration, good times, and exciting people. Students may take some time to realize that their Hollywood impression of college is wrong. Hollywood does not portray college as a place to be scared, confused, overwhelmed, and make mistakes. Students may experience these feelings and worry that they are not normal because what they are experiencing contradicts what they were taught as children. Parents can help by understanding that the ups and downs of college life are an essential part of their child's development and by providing support and encouragement to help their child understand this as well.

Be Prepared for Change

Your student will transform. College and the experiences it provides can impact social, vocational, and personal behavior and choices. It's natural, unavoidable, and can be motivating. However, it is frequently a pain in the neck. You can't stop change, and you may never understand it, but accepting it is within your power and to your and your student's advantage. Remember that your son or daughter will be the same person you sent away to school.

Be Informed About Campus Resources

Use the university's website or their parent calendar and handbook. These resources are geared toward parents and contain a wealth of information about the university and its departments. The best way to mentor your college student throughout the transition to adulthood is by helping them navigate the university by referring them to the appropriate resources. By serving as a reference, you can demonstrate your interest in your student's university life while empowering your student to solve their problems.

Dealing With Their Separation Anxiety

Being concerned about your child when they leave the house is natural. You only know what your child will share with you as he enters college. A parent's anxiety becomes a problem when that parent cannot let go. While we frequently believe that our concern is for another person, in this case, the child, it may be about how you, as the parent, are doing. Will you be okay now that your child has left home?

Parents may struggle with giving up control. It is critical to let go and allow your children to make their own decisions. While you can offer advice and direction, you must take a step back. So, how can parents manage their anxieties while encouraging their children to explore the world without them? Here are some strategies to consider.

Refocus your efforts. You now have more time to devote to yourself and your hobbies. Rekindle old passions. Find out about new ones. Rethink your expectations. Your child will always require your assistance. Your relationship will change as your child matures and gains equal footing. Recognizing this and encouraging a shift in your dynamic will result in more positive interactions and engagement.

When your anxiety is at its peak, it's easy to over-engage and over-extend yourself, doing everything you can for your child, even if that's not what your child requires. Provide advice and direction without putting anyone under pressure. It's a fine line that you must negotiate with your child.

Expect your child to make mistakes. College is a time of discovery for students. It is a time for children to grow apart from their parents and become more self-sufficient. Students will make mistakes as part of the learning process, and parents must prepare for this.

Dealing With Your Own Anxiety

Here's a survival guide to help you as your child adjusts to college life. With these pointers in mind, you'll be able to celebrate your child's departure for college rather than dwell on any feelings of loss.

Prepare for Your Freshman's Departure in Advance

If you're worried about how you'll cope with your children leaving for college, you must be prepared and have made plans for the upcoming change. As a parent, you will grow emotionally and gain much from your child's college experience. You can start a new hobby, a new exercise program, or have a weekly get-together with some of your friends in the weeks leading up to your first-year student's departure.

This is an excellent way to develop the habit of prioritizing your interests and needs before your child leaves for college. It will also make the transition to college feel less drastic. You must mentally prepare for your son's or daughter's departure from college and not avoid thinking about it. While our children are frequently our primary focus and source of energy in our lives, you must figure out how to provide your energy and find new ways to keep yourself busy.

Show Your Support

With your children attending college, you should not feel as if they are about to embark on a new chapter that does not involve you in any way. You will be an essential part of their lives even if you will not live with them full-time. You might even discover that they require you now more than ever. Before the big move, sit down with your child and talk about how you feel about them attending college. It's important to tell your children that you're proud of them and the hard work they've put in to get here but that you'll miss them and want to be as helpful and involved in their college experience as possible.

Take Care of Yourself

If you're having trouble coping with your child leaving for college and leaving your family at home, don't be too hard on yourself. Many parents experience empty nest syndrome, as it is now commonly referred to. Don't feel silly or guilty if you're sad or missing your child. While you're happy for them, it's natural to miss them and wish they were still at home with you.

Parents can't help but worry about their children, even when they know they're safe and making the right choices. However, remember that you raised them well and taught them the life lessons they need to navigate their way through the adult world. You may eventually embrace your empty nest status and embark on home improvement projects you've always wanted to try. Remember how much fun and growth you had when you were his age! It's fantastic for your child to have a similar or even better college experience.

Accept Technology

You can communicate as if your child is in the next room, no matter how far away they are. Thanks to technological advancements in recent years, you no longer have to worry about going weeks or even months without seeing your child once they start college. Your child will always be on the other end of your cell phone. Be prepared for early-morning phone calls asking how to make eggs or late-night texts asking how to use the washing machine and dryer whether your child is attending college in-state, across the country, or even abroad! Technology is a powerful connection tool.

Make Plans for Family Visits

Making plans with your child in advance is a great way to deal with them going to college. You don't have to stop spending time with them just because they don't live with you anymore. While this may be more difficult if they attend a college that is a long distance away, you may be surprised at the variety of visit opportunities. Don't just show up on campus during the school year without informing your child; instead, make plans to visit them during their college's "family weekend" visits. This is an excellent opportunity to visit your child's college and spend time with them.

CONCLUSION

Parents must talk to their teens about puberty, sexuality, sexual orientation, and hygiene. You must find time to have important discussions about these topics with your teen before and when they leave for college.

School is a different environment for teens where they may come face to face with bullies. You must talk to your child about how not to be bullied or bully other children. Teens must acknowledge the importance of maintaining good hygiene and avoiding drugs and alcohol. Male teens must respect females to foster a fulfilling love relationship in the future.

Finding time to talk with your teen about life's challenges and how to prepare for college saves them from depression and anxiety. Now that you've read this book, you are all set to handle the high waters of your teenager so that they can face the challenges of this age confidently.

If this book has helped you talk to your teenager a bit better than a few mumbles here and there, then please leave a review. I'd love to hear about your experiences.

If this book has helped you understand yourself better, please leave a review.

REFERENCES

5 Parenting Tips To Help Your Child Get More Exercise. (n.d.). Retrieved December 3, 2022, from Child Development Institute website:

Aditi, Prerna. (2019, November 23). 6 Reasons Why Some Parents May Fail To Understand Emotional Needs Of Their Kids. Retrieved from https://www.boldsky.com website:

American Academy of Pediatrics. (2018, November 5). What's the Best Way to Discipline My Child? Retrieved from HealthyChildren.org website:

Barnes-Clay, T. (2020, February 15). Parenting through the pain of teenage heartache. Retrieved December 3, 2022, from FQ Magazine website:

Better Health Channel. (2012). Parenting children through puberty. Retrieved from Vic.gov.au website:

Better Health Channel. (2018a, November 5). Teenagers and Sleep. Retrieved from Vic.gov.au website:

Better Health Channel. (2018b, November 5). Teenagers and Sleep. Retrieved from Vic.gov.au website:

Brink, A. (2021, June 14). How to Teach Your Teenager Respect: 5 Practical Steps. Retrieved December 3, 2022, from iMOM website:

Counseling Adolescents About Contraception. (n.d.). Retrieved from www.acog.org website:

Cruz, Mario, MD,, and Ashanti, Nova. (n.d.). Dos and Don'ts when talking to your kids about puberty. Retrieved December 3, 2022, from https://www.inquirer.com website:

Dabkowska, M., Araszkiewicz, A., Dabkowska, A., & Wilkosc, M. (2011). Separation Anxiety in Children and Adolescents. In *www.intechopen.com*. IntechOpen. Retrieved from

Dealing With Your Distant Teen - Troubled Teens. (2019). Retrieved from

Familydoctor.org editorial staff. (2010, June 16). For Parents: Eating Disorders in Teens. Retrieved from familydoctor.org website:

Hartstein, J. (2017). Managing Your Separation Anxiety as Your Child Enters College. Retrieved from US News & World Report website:

Harvard Health Publishing. (2011, March 7). The adolescent brain: Beyond raging hormones - Harvard Health. Retrieved from Harvard Health website:

Health, A. A. (2013, June 25). When is the right time to talk about puberty? Retrieved December 3, 2022, from health enews website:

Healthy Eating During Adolescence. (2015). Retrieved from Johns Hopkins Medicine website:

Hock, E., Eberly, M., Bartle-Haring, S., Ellwanger, P., & Widaman, K. F. (2001). Separation Anxiety in Parents of Adolescents: Theoretical Significance and Scale Development. *Child Development*, *72*(1), 284–298. Retrieved from

How Can Parents Help Teens to Develop Healthy Eating Habits? (n.d.). Retrieved from

How Parents Can Teach Adolescents Responsibility | Psychology Today. (n.d.). Retrieved from www.psychologytoday.com website:

How to Be a Hygienic Teenage Girl: 9 Steps (with Pictures). (n.d.). Retrieved from wikiHow website:

How to Cope With an Emotionally Distant Child. (n.d.). Retrieved from Empowering Parents website:

How to Stay Close to Your Distant Teen. (2014a, February 10). Retrieved December 3, 2022, from Parenthetical website:

How to Stay Close to Your Distant Teen. (2014b, February 10). Retrieved December 3, 2022, from Parenthetical website:

How to Talk with Your Kids About Puberty. (2015). Retrieved from Nationwidechildrens.org website:

How to Teach Your Teen Good Hygiene. (n.d.). Retrieved from Verywell Family website:

How to teach your teenager about consent - ReachOut Parents. (n.d.). Retrieved from parents.au.reachout.com website:

Johns Hopkins Medicine. (2019). The Growing Child: Adolescent 13 to 18 Years. Retrieved from John Hopkins medicine website:

Kids, B. (2016, April 19). The Benefits of Giving Children Responsibilities Rock and Roll Daycare - Best of Boston 2017 - Infant, Toddler, PreK. Retrieved from Rock and Roll Daycare website:

Levy, MD, MPH, S., & Sundaram, BA, S. (2018, August 16). Teens and drugs: 5 tips for talking with your kids. Retrieved from Harvard Health website:

Martha. (2021, December 24). 5 Most Beneficial Hygiene Tips for Teenage Boys. Retrieved December 3, 2022, from Sanjeev Datta Personality School website:

Mathis, M. (2018, October 27). Bullying Prevention: How to Talk So Teens Will Listen. Retrieved December 3, 2022, from We Are Teachers website:

Mayo Clinic Staff. (2018). Healthy body image: Tips for guiding girls. Retrieved from Mayo Clinic website:

Miranda. (2019, October 16). 12 Mom Tested Tips on How to Make Your Teenager Responsible. Retrieved December 3, 2022, from The Reluctant Cowgirl website:

Morin, LCSW, A., & T. Lockhart, PsyD, ABPP, A.-L. (2021, January 31). 5 Ways to Raise an Independent Teen and a Responsible Adult. Retrieved from Verywell Family website:

Morin, LCSW, A., T. Lockhart, PsyD, ABPP, A.-L., & Scherr, R. (2022, June 6). How to Address Kids' Behavior Problems Effectively With Consequences. Retrieved from Verywell Family website:

Nuss-Warren, D. (2021, February 8). Personal Hygiene Habits To Teach Your Son, By Age. Retrieved December 3, 2022, from Moms website:

Office of Population Affairs. (2022). Healthy Relationships in Adolescence | HHS Office of Population Affairs. Retrieved from opa.hhs.gov website:

Parenting, Sexual Orientation and Gender Identity - Family Planning. (n.d.). Retrieved from www.familyplanning.org.nz website:

Personal Hygiene Tips for Tween Girls. (n.d.). Retrieved December 3, 2022, from Verywell Family website:

Philadelphia, T. C. H. (2020, June 25). Talking to Kids about Gender and Sexual Orientation. Retrieved from www.chop.edu website:

Pietro, S. (2016, February 20). Parents Guide to Teenagers and Sleep. Retrieved from Child Mind Institute website:

Pontz, E. (2018, September 4). Creating Safe Boundaries for Teens to Push Against. Retrieved December 3, 2022, from Center for Parent and Teen Communication website:

Powell-Lunder, J. (2013, September 25). Hunkering Down In Her Room: A Rite of Passage or a Cause for Concern? Your Teen Mag. Retrieved December 3, 2022, from Your Teen Magazine website:

Puberty: Your Brain on Hormones. (n.d.). Retrieved from Frontiers for Young Minds website:

Responsibilities Teens Should Be Doing Independently. (2020, February 17). Retrieved from Middle Earth website:

Ross, Kelly Mae, & Moody, J. (2020). 10 Ways to Help Your Teen With the College Decision. Retrieved from US News & World Report website:

Seaton, J. (2019, August 27). The Magic and Science of First Love - Your Teen Mag. Retrieved from Your Teen Magazine website:

Shifting responsibility to your child: teenage years. (2018, May 3). Retrieved from Raising Children Network website:

Smith, M, M.A., M., Robinson, L., Segal, Ph.D., J., & Reid, S. (2018, December 20).. HelpGuide.org. Retrieved from HelpGuide.org website:

Stanford Children's Health. (2019). Retrieved from Stanfordchildrens.org website:

Stanford Children's Health. (2019). The Growing Child: Teenager (13 to 18 Years). Retrieved from Stanfordchildrens.org website:

Stilwell, S. (2022, February 22). Parents Play a Critical Role in Helping Teens with Eating Disorders. Retrieved from AIM Youth Mental Health website:

Talking to your teen about alcohol. (2017). Talking to your teen about alcohol. Retrieved October 30, 2019, from DrinkWise Australia website:

Teaching Teen Accountability & Responsibility. (n.d.). Retrieved December 3, 2022, from Empowering Parents website:

Tips for talking to your kids about sexual orientation. (n.d.). Retrieved from www.childrensmercy.org website:

Tynan-Wood, C. (2022, November 18)). When boys go silent. Retrieved December 3, 2022, from Parenting website:

Unicef. (n.d.). How to talk to your children about bullying. Retrieved from www.unicef.org website:

What are some common teenage responsibilities? (2011, April 1). Retrieved from HowStuffWorks website:

What should I teach my high school-aged teen about pregnancy and reproduction? (n.d.). Retrieved from www.plannedparenthood.org website:

Why boundaries matter... and how to create them! (n.d.). Retrieved December 3, 2022, from The World Needs More Love Letters website:

Wong, A. (2019, September 23). How College Changes the Parent-Child Relationship. Retrieved from The Atlantic website:

www.ingramcontent.com/pod-product-compliance
Lightning Source LLC
Chambersburg PA
CBHW011223120626
46545CB00010B/3134